THE JOY OF INTELLIGENT FASTING

*.....For the first time a book that deals with the **physical, mental, and spiritual** benefits of fasting.....*

by DR. FREDERICK A. HOGAN

GROWTH AND CHANGE PUBLISHING
P.O.BOX 647
OKEMOS, MI. 48805

ISBN:0-7392-0112-3
Library of Congress Catalog Card Number: 99-94054

ALL SCRIPTURE QUOTATIONS FROM KJV OR NIV

Morris Publishing
3212 East Highway 30
Kearney, NE 68847
1-800-650-7888

CONTENTS

Acknowledgments

Thanks to God who has given me the strength to endure the hardships of life and remain in his will. Thanks to Eugene and Rosalie who showed by example the importance of a consistent prayer life. Thanks to the membership at Growth and Change Christian Community Church for their prayers and support, And thanks to Noelle, Frederick II , and Daniel who have made my life worth the journey.

Pastor Hogan

FORWARD

Dr. Hogan is an amazing man. He holds his medical degree and has enjoyed a successful, prospering practice for a number of years now. Even while seeing upwards to forty patients a day, Dr. Hogan still made time to attend Bible College in the evenings to earn yet another degree; this one in theology. And today he has even made time to launch a powerful new church which focuses on genuine relationship with God.

Dr. Hogan is refreshing. Here is a medical doctor with a heart distinctly committed to drawing into the presence of God the Father and motivating others to do so as well. I love this dear brother. When I'm with Dr. Hogan, my heart burns within me. I somehow feel that I'm in the presence of one who really knows Jesus intimately.

In *The Joy of Intelligent Fasting*, you'll find some authoritative biblical truths concerning the discipline of fasting. Yet beyond that, Dr. Hogan gives you some very practical help in your fasting adventure by getting right down "where the rubber meets the road." Don't think you'll be the same after reading this book. You won't. You will be changed forever when you take that step of faith and begin to apply the plan this book lays out for you.

Who needs this book? Here are just a few of the "who's" that came to mind as I read through *The Joy of Intelligent Fasting*:

Every pastor and church worker
Every person who needs direction from God
Every person beginning a new ministry

Every person who wants to impact his or her generation
Every person who needs more energy
Every person who needs to be delivered from a nasty habit
Every husband, every wife, every couple, every single person
Every person seeking God for a marriage partner
Every person desiring victory over demonic influence
Every person who needs added spiritual power
Every person experiencing the pain of depression and anxiety
Every person needing a breakthrough (relationally, socially, mentally, financially)
Every person desiring to live a long and fruitful life
Every parent who cares about children
Every church member who is thinking about leaving church
Every person facing a new job opportunity

The list could go on, but I think you get the point. It's very obvious, I'm sure, by now that you can see we all need this book. I know that as you read these pages and begin to practice the joy of intelligent fasting as I have, your whole life will enter a new and fresh dimension that you've never even dreamed about.

When you've finished reading a chapter, you'll be able to get a quick recap with Dr. Hogan's "Points to Remember" found at the close of each chapter.

You may want to copy these "Points to Remember" pages and carry them with you as you practice the miracle discipline of fasting. Read them over often until you can remember these important points and even share them with others. And get ready for a life-changing adventure as you thrust forth into.....

.....*The Joy of Intelligent Fasting!*

Dave Williams , Pastor
Mount Hope Church
Lansing, Michigan

Introduction

Fasting has caused quite a controversy in the Body of Christ. Some Christians regard fasting as a waste of time. Many believe it is a futile exercise while, others fast whenever they feel like it. Fasting is the missing link Christians need to move into the perfect will of God and become like Christ in this world. On the surface the word of God does not offer much instruction on fasting, but taking a closer look in the Bible there are many scriptures which refer to fasting and people who fasted. This book attempts to answer such questions as:

Why and when should we fast? What does fasting accomplish? What should we do and avoid during a fast? The role God plays in fasting and whether He approves of it. What are important facts to know about fasting?

Before anyone endeavors to go on a fast, he should educate himself about fasting. Many people fast without knowing much about it. For such people, the main concern becomes the spiritual benefits of fasting. When fasting results in physical and emotional breakdown, it diminishes the spiritual gain. Man is a triune being -- body, soul and spirit. When the body and soul are neglected during a fast, it becomes impossible to make an optimal spiritual gain. This neglect reduces the fast to nothing more than starving for God.

This book also focuses on how long a fast should be and what to consume during a fast. Many people make the mistake of going on a dry fast, which means abstinence from food and drink. Dry fasts may work well for one day, but beyond that, a person should at least drink water. This book discusses how to benefit physically, emotionally and spiritually from a fast. I do not believe anyone should go on a fast without understanding that there are physical, emotional and spiritual benefits to fasting. A great number of members of the body of Christ fast because of the spiritual gain, neglecting the emotional and physical benefits. They talk about the many wonderful things that happen in their lives as a result of fasting. Why then, are there not more Christians fasting? I can attribute that to four reasons:

Ignorance: Many Christians do not understand what happens physically, emotionally and spiritually when one is deprived of food. Many will fast without any clear reasons. Not much is being taught in our churches about fasting and you can only practice what you know. As a result, many Christians do not understand what wonderful benefits there are when we fast and pray.

Unpleasant experience: Most Christians enjoy eating, which makes fasting a very unpleasant physical experience. Some also fast for long periods without water, which makes fasting even more unpleasant. Fasting will allow Christians to understand the power of the flesh and it's controlling power over their lives. It will also allow them to know that the Greater One in us has power over the flesh.

Lack of understanding of God's Will: God's Will (purpose and plan) for our lives can only be realized when

2

we are sensitive enough to understand, what He communicates. God communicates to us through His Word, His leaders, prayer, praise, and quiet time before Him. Fasting generates the sensitivity to God like nothing else.

No specific directions about fasting in the Bible: What the Bible says about fasting is quite generic. It leaves the length of time and how often we should fast up to us. What the Bible highlights in all instances of fasting is that those individuals fasting are focused on God.

Chapter One

The Significance of Fasting

Fasting has been practiced for thousands of years. For centuries, almost all world religions have observed fasting as a religious duty. Only recently have Christians truly understood the spiritual, emotional and physical benefits of fasting. Some Christians have reaped the spiritual benefits from fasting, although not many have tried to focus on the emotional and physical benefits.

The word "fast" in Hebrew is **SUM**, which means **TO COVER THE MOUTH** or **TO AFFLICT THE SOUL**. In ancient times, fasting was done primarily as a superstitious gesture to appease the gods. People felt that the gods were jealous of the pleasures of men and when men could purposely suffer through fasting, it would appease the gods. Fasting was like a peace sacrifice to the gods. Ancient men attributed to the gods the same thought processing potential as man. We now understand that God does not think like man at all. Fasting benefits man more than it does Almighty God.

Ezra 8:21: *"Then I proclaimed a fast there, at the river of Ahava, that we might afflict ourselves before our God ..."*

Fasting implies the sacrifice of the personal will in order to better understand God's Will. The gains are personal. This does not imply that a person cannot go on a corporate fast. Even in a corporate setting like a church community, fasting remains a personal commitment between the individual and God. The decision to go on a fast, and its duration, should be left up to the individual. Even in a corporate setting, fasting is very personal. Although the corporate body benefits from the fast, the individual benefits personally. In essence, the fast is between the individual and God. It is the same as when we stand with others to worship God. Even though there are many, worship is between the individual worshipper and God.

Fasting with prayer, worship and praise leaves man unencumbered with earthly matters, which is the key. This enables man to devote himself, with less distractions, to God. Sincere devotion to God guarantees greater sensitivity to Him. When a person abstains from food, the physical body rests from trying to maintain itself by digesting food. By the same token, abstinence from negative stimuli that enter the soul through the senses rests the emotions. With the physical and emotional rest, the spirit readily opens to God, becoming more sensitive to commune with God.

Regular fasting brings the believer to a more sensitive relationship with the Almighty God. The benefits of fasting are paramount. One cannot begin to understand what happens to an individual who decides to deny himself and begin to fast before God. Believers need to fast more intelligently than they have before. In the past, people fasted blindly because there was very little teaching on the subject. Sometimes people decided to fast for very personal reasons. Prayer, worship and praise are an integral part of any fast.

Nehemiah 9:3 endorses this: *"And they stood up in their place and read in the book of the law of the Lord their God one fourth of the day; and another fourth part they confessed, and worshipped the Lord their God."* The scripture above relates a certain pattern they followed while fasting.

King David also reveals the power of praise:

"Still the enemy and the avenger;" **Psalm 8:2**

"Execute vengeance upon the heathen, and punishment upon the people;

To bind their kings with chains, and their nobles with fetters of iron;

To execute upon them the judgment written: this honour have all His saints. Praise ye the Lord." **Psalm 149:7-9**

That is why David exhorts believers to come into his gates with thanksgiving and praise, **Psalm 100:4-5.** What gives fasting its value is the sacrifice of one's personal will. David calls it the *"humbling of the soul"* in **Psalm 35:12.** When a person can `will' to eat, but lays aside that will in favor of going before God, ministering to Him with praise, worship and prayer, that is personal sacrifice. There is

6

much to be gained from such an attitude towards fasting. When talking about those who will fast according to God's guidelines, Isaiah says: *"... and I will cause thee to ride upon the high places of the earth, and feed thee with the heritage of Jacob thy father; for the mouth of the Lord has spoken."* **Isaiah 58:14** The value is not in what benefits God, but what benefits the person who is willing to make the sacrifice. Such a fast is an act of deepest humility before God.

Points to Remember

- Fasting means afflicting the soul in order to gain physically, emotionally and spiritually. **(Ezra 8:21)**

- There is an individual fast where one person decides to go on a fast. There is also a corporate fast where a group of people decide to fast together.

- Always accompany fasting with prayer, praise, worship and reading the Word. **(Nehemiah 9:3)**

- Praise is a weapon to silence the devil. **(Psalm 8:2; Psalm 149:4-9)**

- Fasting is an act of humility before God. David refers to it as the humbling of the soul. **(Psalm 35:13)**

- Fasting gives physical and emotional rest.

- It makes the believer more sensitive to God.

- People should fast more intelligently.

Chapter Two

Benefits of Biblical Fasting

Since fasting has to be a personal decision, it is far more beneficial for individuals to search the scriptures themselves. We are going to look at some scriptures that pertain to fasting. For the benefit of those who are not well-versed about fasting, this book will attempt to be a Bible study manual on fasting. Note that the scriptures will be given in part. For better understanding, please go back and read the whole chapter from which the quotation was taken.

The Biblical guidelines for fasting are outlined in **Leviticus 16:29:** *"And this shall be a statute forever unto you, that in the seventh month, on the tenth day of the month, ye shall afflict your souls and do no work at all, whether it be one of your own country, or a stranger that sojourneth among you."*

In **Isaiah 58**, God accused His people of doing what they pleased during the fast. They did not fast like the Ninevites **(Jonah 3:7)**. During the fast they were still ruled by their fleshly desires.

"... Behold, in the day of your fast ye find pleasure, and exact all your labours.

Behold, ye fast for strife and debate, and to smite with the fist of wickedness: ye shall not fast as ye do this day, to make your voice heard from on high." (Isaiah 58:3-4)

Isaiah 58 is the most popular and well-read scripture on fasting. Verse 6 reads: *"Is this not the fast that I have chosen, to loose the bands of wickedness, to undo the heavy burdens, to let the oppressed go free and that ye break every yoke."*

In this scripture, the Lord points out four things that could potentially happen when a believer fasts:

Loose the bands of wickedness;
Undo heavy burdens;
Let the oppressed go free;
Break every yoke.

LOOSE THE BANDS OF WICKEDNESS

Many of the people in Biblical times had a tendency to stray away from God and indulge in all kinds evil practices. This is what the Lord addresses when He talks about the bands of wickedness. These evil practices led the people to indulge in the wickedness of foreign idol worship.

Jezebel, a foreigner who became the wife of King Ahab, brought idol gods which caused the people of God to stray from the path of righteousness. In **I Kings 21:12**, Jezebel proclaimed a fast, plotting to dispossess Naboth of his vineyard by killing him. The Lord obviously opposes such attitudes of wickedness during a fast. Remember that the Jewish culture came from God. The word *"culture"* comes from a Latin word *"colere"* meaning *"worship"*. Fasting was one of the basic elements of Jewish culture. It was meant to afflict the soul while enriching the spirit.

10

This tendency still prevails in some circles in the modern church. People start very innocently playing games which have a negative spiritual significance in their original cultural setting, like the ouija board, or dungeons and dragons. After a while, this grows into an area of major interest, becoming a driving force, like an addiction, in a person's life.

On the other hand, Esther fasted according to God's pattern, pleading with God concerning the imminent annihilation of the Jews. **(Esther 4:16)** This humbling was responsible for the Jews coming out of the danger not only unscathed, but also with the wealth of those who wanted to spoil them. Jehosaphat experienced similar results in **II Chronicles 20**.

UNDO HEAVY BURDENS

Christians easily get preoccupied with the cares and burdens of life. People who fall into this category usually worry about areas that God has already promised to take care of. Major areas of concern are family; ministry (God's work); and finances. This is what the Lord says about:

FAMILY:
"And all thy children shall be taught of the Lord; and great shall be the peace of thy children." (Isaiah 54:13)

"... for I will contend with him that contended with thee, and I will save thy children." (Isaiah 49:25b)

Satan has launched an all-out attack on the family. He usually tries to focus on the weakest link, whether it be a child, mom or dad. When he attacks one member, life for the entire family becomes more difficult.

11

Instead of happiness and joy that should exist, family life becomes a burden.

MINISTRY:

"I took you from the ends of the earth, from the farthest corners I called you. I said, `You are my servant.' I have chosen you and have not rejected you.

So do not fear, for I am with you; do not be dismayed, for I am your God. I will strengthen you and help you; I will uphold you with my righteous right hand." **(Isaiah 41:9-10)**

Ministry work should be easiest to do because it is God's work, but for some it is becoming increasingly more difficult. This usually happens when we forget that it is His ministry and not ours. It will take His strength, His ideas and His long suffering for us to do His will.

FINANCES:

"Let your conversation be without covetousness; and be content with such things as ye have; for He hath said, I will never leave thee, nor forsake thee.

So that we may boldly say, The Lord is my helper, and I will not fear what man shall do unto me." **(Hebrews 13:5-6)**

There never seems to be enough money for everything we want to do. The burden of debt is real, and very humbling. Most people in debt become preoccupied with debt, trying to pay it off. Some may even take an extra job, leaving less time to do anything for God. If we look around, we will find that much of our debt stems from wants rather than needs.

Undoing heavy burdens does not necessarily mean that they will actually disappear. Fasting enables us to rest physically and emotionally, thus detaching ourselves from carnal situations. Our burden may still exist, but if our focus is on God, the burden becomes less important and so much easier to bear.

TO LET THE OPPRESSED GO FREE

In **Isaiah 1:17**, God gives a command: *"Learn to do well; seek judgment, relieve the oppressed, judge the fatherless, plead for the widow."*

In **Amos 4:1-2**, the Lord decrees a judgment against those who oppress His people: *"Hear ye this word, ye kine of Bashan, that are in the mountain of Samaria, which oppress the poor, which crush the needy, which say to their masters, Bring, and let us drink.*

The Lord God hath sworn by His holiness, that, lo, the days shall come upon you, that he will take you away with hooks, and your posterity with fishhooks."

During a fast, the Lord expected the people to deal generously with the poor who were in their houses. Since they expected unmerited favor from God, they had to give the same favor to those under their rule. **(Isaiah 58:7)** When a nation was under any kind of oppression, the civil leaders would call for a fast. As the people called out to God by reason of their oppression, He would miraculously come and deliver, as He says in **Isaiah 58:8-9:**

"Then shall thy light break forth as the morning, and thine health shall spring forth speedily; and thy righteousness shall go before thee; the glory of the Lord shall be thy reward.

13

Then thou shall call and the Lord shall answer; thou shall cry and He shall say, Here I am. If thou take from the midst of thee the yoke, the putting forth of the finger, and speaking vanity."
Modern-day oppression for the Christian is usually in the form of someone controlling another. Sometimes it is a group of people being controlled and manipulated in the name of God by a charismatic leader. Fear plays an important role because most members of the group feel that God will somehow not bless them or will not love them if they leave the group. When these leaders call a fast, the focus is not on God, but on themselves. Fasting will allow the individual to focus on God and not on the godlike leader. Then God can speak to them about this ungodly control. Fasting, according to God's guidelines, will let the oppressed go free.

AND THAT YE BREAK EVERY YOKE
The yoke referred to is the yoke of bondage. From time to time the people of God were faced with imminent invasion by the enemy. **(2 Chronicles 20)** In **Isaiah 10,** Judah faced oppression by the Assyrians. Fasting increases the anointing in a believer's life. The people of Judah went on a fast and increased their anointing. To anoint someone was to separate them for a special office or task God wanted them to fulfill. This anointing also gave them special ability to accomplish the task. With the increased anointing (fatness according to the Amplified version), yokes are destroyed. **(Isaiah 10:27)**
Oppression by an enemy would be equated to bondage by demonic spirits.

14

In **Isaiah 58**, the Lord primarily addresses a people who had been wrapped and tied up into activities which caused them to serve other gods. Fasting, according to God's guidelines, increased the glory of God in their lives and destroyed the yoke of oppression.

Points to Remember

- There are certain guidelines to be observed during a fast. **(Leviticus 16:29)**

- Fasting is not a time for the people to do as they please. It is a time devoted to God. **(Isaiah 58:3b)**

- Fasting will loose the bands of wickedness; undo heavy burdens; let the oppressed go free; break every yoke. **(Isaiah 58:6)**

- Intermingling with foreign cultures, caused the people to do what was offensive to God during a fast. Jezebel called a fast, during which she plotted to kill Naboth. **(I Kings 21:12)**

- Esther's fast broke the power of oppression and freed the people of God. **(Esther 4:16)**

- God has promised to take care of our families **(Isaiah 54:13)**, our ministries **(Isaiah 41:9-10)** and our finances **(Hebrews 13:5-6)**.

- During the Lord's fast, the yoke of oppression had to be loosed. **(Isaiah 58:7)**

- Fasting according to Biblical principles increased the anointing and destroyed the yoke. **(Isaiah 10:27)**

16

Chapter Three

Cleansing the Temple

"Know ye not that ye are the temple of God, and that the spirit of God dwelleth in you? If any man defile the temple of God, him shall God destroy; for the temple of God is holy, which ye are." **I Corinthians 3:16-17**

If the human body is the temple of God, then like all temples it needs regular cleansing. There are so many things that can defile the temple. A house or an apartment closed for two or three months gets dirty, without anyone occupying it. Dust has a way of settling everywhere, even in closed houses.

FOOD AS A CONTAMINANT

"Life is a tragedy of nutrition. Man digs his grave with a knife and fork." **(Paul Bragg)**

This saying may be trite but true. Modern man is constantly stuffing his body with food, never giving it any time to rest. Food has nutrients, but much of our modern day food has impurities. Not only do our bodies have to assimilate what is good, but also detoxify and get rid of what causes contamination. It takes a great deal of the body energy to carry out this process with any efficiency because most of the processed food is full of contaminants. Fasting gives the body time to rest from this never ending process and to cleanse itself.

The greatest tragedy in modern civilization is that some people die from gluttony while others die from lack of food. Paul equates gluttony with idolatry.

"For many walk, of whom I have told you often, and now tell you even in weeping, that they are enemies of the cross of Christ: Whose end is destruction, whose God is their belly, and whose glory is in their shame, who mind earthly things" **Philippians 3:18-19**

The media once did an investigative documentary report on hot dogs, sausages and cold cuts. The report revealed that some of the meat in the market had a percentage of rodent hair. In response, people stopped buying hot dogs for about a month. After some time the sales went up again. Many times people eat contaminants unaware. Whether ignorant or informed, when contaminants are consumed, they have a negative effect on the body. Although the people who bought hot dogs were ignorant of rodent contamination, it still affected their health.

Because of contaminants in the food, the body carries toxins that need elimination. Health experts agree that almost all sickness can be traced to diet. On a normal day the human body is barraged with non-foods like sodium, processed sugar, artificial sweeteners, food coloring, preservatives, and pesticides found in most store-bought food. To eliminate these toxins, the body needs rest. The three meals prescribed daily do not give the body the proper rest between meals to heal itself. Some of this refined food lacks natural fiber (which aids in elimination) causing the digestive tract to be sluggish. This affects the whole body making it difficult to function properly.

Everything that God created has the potential to heal and renew itself. The same applies for the human body. Fasting gives the body time to rest so that it can heal itself. The energy that would be used by digestion is used to cleanse the body by eliminating toxins that could potentially affect major organs.

A normal body needs regular cleansing. Some experts recommend twenty-four hours weekly. During a one-day cleansing fast it is beneficial to drink an abundance of distilled water. Six to eight glasses daily will help eliminate toxins.

For a person who has never fasted, I recommend several twenty-four hour fasts before trying a longer fast. During a fast, hunger pangs are just a reminder that man's main sustenance is God. *"... that he might know that man doth not live by bread only, but by every word that proceedeth out of the mouth of the Lord, doth man live."* **Deuteronomy 8:5** During a cleansing fast remember to draw closer to God in prayer, worship and studying the Word. This increases strength and resistance, and makes fasting a meaningful and fruitful time.

SOULISH CONTAMINANTS
"I will set no wicked thing before my eyes: I hate the work of them that turn aside; it shall not cleave to me." **Psalm 101:3**

Contamination does not only come from food, but also from what we do, we say, what we watch on television and in the movies, and what we think about. All these can defile the temple. In the 1950s, a group of experts conducted an experiment on subliminal suggestion. They went into a movie show and flashed on the screen where everybody could see, "EAT POPCORN, DRINK COKE." They flashed it so quickly that nobody in the movie theater knew about it except the people doing the experiment. The sale of popcorn and Coke increased by a considerable percentage as a result of the experiment.

By the same token, watching television has adversely affected society. An hour of watching TV may expose us to several scenes of adultery, illicit sex, promiscuity and murder, which have adverse effects on the soul of the person watching. Some Christians feel that because they are born again, the violence and filth have no effect on them, but it can and does defile the soul. Sit-coms and soap operas have sexual inferences, innuendoes, connotations, undertones, dirty jokes and coarse joking, which the Bible clearly says should be avoided.

"But fornication and all uncleanness, or covetousness, let it not be once named among you, as becometh saints. Neither filthiness, nor foolish talking, nor jesting, which are not convenient, but rather giving of thanks." **Ephesians 5:4**

Christians need to be very careful because some of the TV entertainment may not only be dirty, but simply unholy. The effects on the soul from viewing such vicarious experiences on TV are the same as if they were true life experiences. Whatever a person does, says, watches and thinks about may poison the soul. After a while, the effects of these experiences call for the restoration of the soul.

In a physical sense, the liver is the detoxifying organ. It clears out most poisons that are ingested. Detoxification is a process by which the liver breaks down contaminants in order to discard and render them harmless to the body. Abstaining from television during a fast cuts off the constant supply of toxins that comes through the senses and into the soul. Prayer, praise, worship and feeding on the Word of God during this period renews the mind and restores the soul.

I Corinthians 6:19-20: *"What? Know ye not that your body is the temple of the Holy Ghost which is in you, which ye have of God, and ye are not your own? You are bought with a price: therefore, glorify the Lord in your body, and in your spirit, which are God's."*

The body as the temple of the Holy Spirit can be kept clean through fasting. As in the case of contaminated hot dogs, filth can enter an unsuspecting person's physical body. Likewise, filth can enter an unsuspecting person's mind through subliminal suggestions on a movie screen or through watching television. What we eat, hear or watch on television can damage us physically, emotionally and spiritually.

Some Christians go to sleep leaving the television set on through the night. The most devilish programs and commercials are aired after midnight. The soul, which never sleeps, is exposed to all kinds of wickedness while the body sleeps. This results in soulish contamination, creating the need to fast regularly in order to cleanse the temple. Without regular cleansing these contaminants can become permanent fixtures in our temples, resulting in anxiety, depression and even physical sickness.

Unfortunately, a number of people go for years without fasting. Regular fasting begins a pattern that can make fasting as easy as breathing. Believers ought to fast regularly. In some circles fasting has lost its meaning. The majority of churchgoers do it because everyone else in church does it.

A weekly twenty-four hour fast would break the habit of not fasting and create a fasting routine. Every believer should aim at fasting three days a month. This fast would cleanse the body physically, cleanse the mind emotionally, leaving the spirit clear and unhindered to communicate with God. At the end of the book there are suggested patterns offered for specific times of fasting.

WHEN IN NEED OF PHYSICAL, EMOTIONAL OR SPIRITUAL HEALING

A person suffering from a severe chronic disease should consider fasting.

Severe chronic disease means that the disease has progressed near a life threatening stage, while chronic refers to an ongoing disease, such as diabetes who's symptoms may be mild. When diabetes begins, it is not difficult to manage. After a person has been diabetic for ten or more years, there is a possibility of organ damage, and sometimes organ system damage, such as eyes, kidneys, and blood vessels. This can be severe. When these start taking their toll, there arises a need for some physical healing, and sometimes also emotional healing. In such a case, the patient needs to hear from God. Fasting will bring the person closer to God, to hear His voice and instruction.

Breaking food down for assimilation involves several organs and a large amount of energy. The moment the chewing of food begins, the brain commands the blood to flow into the intestines to aid with digestion. Different foods take different amounts of time and energy to digest. After a large meal, the brain becomes sluggish because the normal percentage of total blood needed for thought processing is reduced, and for a while a higher percentage is shunted to the digestive tract to facilitate digestion.

In the case of a terminal illness like cancer, sufferers tend to lose weight even though they eat. It seems as though the more cancer victims eat, the more weight they lose. Even though they eat, they lose weight because the nourishment of the tumor seems to take precedence over the body. After the food has passed through the liver into the blood stream, the tumor begins to steal whatever nutrition is available in the blood stream. the cancer grows larger while the host continues to lose weight.

I believe that in some cases the host can starve the cancer by fasting. The more the patient weighs at the start of the fasting period, the better the chance of survival.

Smith Wigglesworth, by the unction of the Holy Spirit, would advise terminal cancer victims to fast. Though it sounded harsh when he proclaimed it, many were healed because the cancer would starve and fall off. Putting aside the plate and searching for the Heart of God concerning terminal illness, would be most beneficial to the victim of any terminal illness. They will need the close supervision of a physician and a Pastor knowledgeable about fasting. Regular fasting can cleanse the body of many impurities before they can cause sickness and disease. Fasting, with prayer, praise, worship and constantly reading the Word is a viable choice for the terminally ill.

DEPRESSION

Depression is an emotional illness that effects both Christians and non Christians. The pressure exerted by the stresses of life can bring about depression. Our schedules are monotonous and never ending and our relationships are strained because of our schedules. Sometimes mild depression is difficult to detect because it usually has a slow onset. If a Christian is depressed, he should fast with worship, prayer and praise to God, seeking a Godly solution to the depression. If he wants to visit a doctor, by all means he should do so.

Pharmaceutical companies have manufactured helpful antidepressants. They all seem to work well.

These drugs are to be taken for a specified period of time, although some patients may require them for long-term use. Most people who have been depressed once will probably be revisited by depression. A Christian suffering from depression has to seek God with fasting and stay on the medication till the answer comes.

STRESS ANXIETY

"Be careful for nothing; but in everything by prayer and supplication, with thanksgiving, let your requests be made known unto God. And the peace of God which passeth all understanding, shall keep your hearts and minds through Christ Jesus." **Philippians 4:6-7**

"Humble yourselves therefore under the might hand of God, that He may exalt you in due time: Casting all your care upon Him; for He careth for you." **I Peter 5:6-7** (Also read the Amplified version.)

Stress and anxiety could result in physical and emotional problems. When a person is exposed to emotional stress, it can begin to take a physical toll on him. There are many physical illnesses that stem from or made worse by emotional stress and anxiety. Type-A individuals thrive with stress and anxiety, always feeling a compulsion to do more and more. This type of behavior can be quite self-destructive.

Christians are not immune to stress. Some will exhibit the type-A behavior in the name of the Lord. Christian leaders who tend to do everything and lay persons who feel the need to perform endless tasks usually end up being stressed out and full of anxiety.

Leaders can become stressed out just trying to keep up with how important they think they are. These individuals need emotional and physical healing. By its ability to purge, fasting can rest the emotions and bring everything into the proper perspective. Fasting, with prayer, praise and worship allows one to hear from God concerning the matter which causes stress anxiety. *"Which of you by taking thought can add one cubit unto his stature? .... But seek first the kingdom of God and His righteousness; and all these things shall be added unto you."* Matthew 6:27,33

SEVERE DEMONIC INFLUENCE

I did not say demon possession because I do not believe that Christians can be demon possessed. Demon possession refers to the spirit man being completely controlled by Satan. A person with Christ as his Lord and Savior cannot be possessed by a demon. Christians suffer from demonic influence, where demons can manifest in the body and/or the soulish realm of human beings who may be born again.

"My sheep listen to my voice; I know them, and they follow me. I give them eternal life, and they shall never perish; no one can snatch them out of my Father's hand. I and the Father are one." John 10:27-30

A person influenced by demons suffers from demonic oppression. Some Christians operate for long periods under demonic influence. For example, there are Christians who struggle with alcoholism, drug abuse, lust and gambling, just to name a few.

Most of these people want to lead good Christian lives, but find themselves yielding to the temptation at the onslaught of severe demonic influences. The demonic influence can be so strong that they can find themselves involved in the sinful lifestyle from time to time. They quickly come to God penitent. Some sincerely hate the sinful ways and want to lead clean Christian lives, but the strong influence of demonic spirits keeps these Christians running back and forth. Satan gives them every opportunity to fall back into that lifestyle by making it easily accessible to them. Fasting breaks the dominance of the flesh (where many demons manifest) and will prepare the Christian for deliverance. Most people are driven into sinful lifestyles because of the physical pleasure the demons demand. Habitual fasting accompanied by prayer, worship and study of the Word, increases spiritual fortitude, which boosts resistance against demonic oppression. I have observed many young men get delivered from drugs by fasting. When the system is clean, it naturally rejects what is unclean. Quitters have testified that after a fast, they tried to smoke again and became nauseated. In my experience, fasting and coming before God can deal with any weakness of the flesh that is associated with demonic influence.

LACK OF MOTIVATION TO LOSE WEIGHT

When there is no motivation to keep the temple fit, or lose weight, go on a fast. You may say, "Doctor Hogan, I cannot lose weight. I have been trying to lose weight for ten years."

Remember, a believer has to keep that temple fit. The Bible says that a believer's body is the temple of the Holy Spirit. His Holy Spirit that was sent to this earth has to have your body as His temple. Some believers are extremely overweight and believe that they cannot lose weight. They confess to everyone that they cannot lose any weight. These are the people who do not keep a disciplined exercise schedule. They buy every piece of equipment advertised on television but because of the lack of discipline, they use it for a week and put it away without getting much benefit from it. After piling up the latest equipment in their closets and basements, they sit, putting the blame on lack of motivation, nerves or the devil. The same group of people usually lack the motivation to eat properly.

Cannot Lose Weight

This problem afflicts many Americans today. It has boosted the weight loss business into being a multi-million dollar business. Some people make plenty of money on other people's inability to lose weight. The same people who contend that they cannot lose weight, do not stop eating. They cannot pass the cakes and pies, and are always attracted to all-you-can-eat restaurants.

• Lack of motivation to keep the temple fit and lose weight may indicate a need to fast.

• If you meet the following profile cycle, you really need to fast.

Try a diet, have short-term success, cheat some, relapse, eat more and gain more weight.

When there is no motivation to keep the temple fit, the person needs to consult God.

First of all, confess your problem to Him. It may be a confession like the following:

Lord, I cannot lose a pound. I have been trying, but I don't have the power to stop eating. I need to lose weight so that I can be a lot healthier. This will make me feel good and cause the people around me to appreciate me more. It may even enhance my marriage. Lord, I need to lose some weight."

When this is the person's plea, there needs to be a decision made to fast, pray and spend time with God on a regular basis. A person fasting to lose weight also needs to repent in certain areas. It is useless to stop eating for a day or two, and go back to the same eating habits that induced the weight gain in the first place. Drastic steps need to follow the decision to lose weight.

• Avoid processed and prepackaged food: TV dinners, cookies, canned food, etc. These foods are loaded with sugar, sodium and other preservatives that have little or no nutritional value.

• Fifty to seventy-five percent of food intake should be raw fruits and vegetables. These are rich in natural fibers and active enzymes. They supply the nutritional needs of the body.

• All meat should be chemical free. This may sound impossible to fulfill. The growth- hormone raised meat sold in supermarkets is not nearly as healthy as organic meat. It may be loaded with growth hormones that can contribute to more weight gain. There are still farms where one can buy chemical-free meat. Organic meat is also available at cooperative stores and health food stores.

If the store does not have it, they can order it.
• Avoid saturated fat.

"Speak to the children of Israel, saying, `Ye shall eat no manner of fat, of ox, or of sheep, or of goat.'"
Leviticus 7:23
• Avoid dairy products, eggs and refined sugar.

Please note that the purpose for fasting is not to lose weight, but to draw strength from God until a disciplined lifestyle is mastered. A few pounds may be lost in the process, but fasting is not an effective means of losing weight, unless you are going to go on a modified fast (chapter 10) for an extended period of time. Those people who suffer severe weight problems should consider going on a modified fast. This modified fast can be followed until the desired weight goal has been achieved. This may take a year or two. Hopefully by the end of that time neither discipline nor weight will be a problem anymore. The person will have cultivated new habits and lost the taste for unwholesome food. When a person cannot lose weight he needs to seek God.

When You Cannot Exercise
Exercise is for everyone, both normal and overweight people. Everyone needs to be on a daily exercise program. Only about 30 percent of Americans exercise regularly, even though regular exercise has proven to be a health benefit. We are chronic eaters in America and exercise would help keep many of us from being overweight. It also helps our circulation, decreasing our chances of a heart attack. Exercise is so beneficial that to neglect it would be an invitation to poor health.

Poor health is not God's will for our lives. When a person cannot exercise, that is another reason to submit to God in fasting. Ask God for the ability to regularly exercise in order to keep the temple fit.

When You Cannot Eat Properly

"Be not among winebibbers and riotous eaters of flesh: For the drunkard and the glutton shall come to poverty." **Proverbs 23:20-21**

This problem affects a high percentage of the population. From early in the socialization process children are taught to eat the "right" food. Meat is the staple food of most Americans, with chicken, beef and pork as the most popular. Most of us in America have been socialized to think that we must include meat with every meal. There are thousands of vegetarians who get more than enough protein through their intake of vegetables. Meat eaters will get enough protein by eating meat only twice a week as long as their diet contains vegetables, fruits and nuts daily. Remember, cattle are a source of much of our protein, and they are vegetarians.

Points to Remember

• Food sold in grocery stores may contain indigestible contaminants. The processing and refining of foods eliminates the fiber necessary for the elimination of waste products in the body.

• As the temple of God the human body needs regular cleansing.

• Health experts agree that all sickness can be traced to food. Fasting gives the body time to rest so that it can heal itself.

• A normal body needs regular cleansing three days a month or one day a week.

• Hunger pangs are a reminder of the power of the flesh and that man's main sustenance is God.

• Secular television contaminates the soul by exposing it to wickedness and promiscuity, likewise the practice of sleeping with the TV on exposes the soul to negative stimuli.

• Because of the inability to differentiate between a true life and vicarious experience, the mind takes every scene portrayed on television as if it were a true life experience. This has a negative effect on the human soul.

• Fasting can benefit people who suffer from chronic illness..

• When the system rests from digesting food, the energy that would be used for the digestion is redirected to healing the body.

• The monotony of life can bring stress that leads to depression. Antidepressants are helpful in reducing the symptoms of depression and fasting has proven to be an effective means for understanding the cause of the depression.

• Fasting can reduce the power of any form of demonic oppression. By breaking the power of the flesh, fasting boosts resistance against demonic pressure preparing the believer for deliverance and making him more sensitive to the voice of God. **John 10:27-30**

Chapter Four

Enhance Fellowship

... WITH GOD

Mark 12:30 *"And thou shalt love the Lord they God with all thy heart, and with all thy soul, and with all thy mind, and with all thy strength: this is the first commandment."*

In this fast paced life we lead, there are many daily activities that bid for attention and time. The amount of energy used by our mere existence, like going to work or taking care of the family, constantly competes with the time that is owed to God. Fasting provides an escape route from this helter-skelter existence in order to regroup and reenergize ourselves. Without a conscious effort to shift focus from life's endless demands, to God, the relationship with God is in jeopardy. A life of disciplined fasting helps to reestablish our priorities.

Fasting must be accompanied by prayer, praise worship and reading the Word of God. This makes fasting more than just a hunger strike. The absence of communion with God during a fast makes it almost impossible for one to know God's priorities for his life. Without the proper priorities man will rationalize his priorities and become involved in the activities he can justify. The digestive system takes a considerable amount of energy to run. After a meal, the body wants to rest. When food reaches the stomach, the blood that would be used by the brain for running the body rushes to the stomach.

This causes a person to be sluggish after a meal because the blood used for thinking is now being used to digest food.

It is much easier to pray when the digestive system rests. With no food to digest, a clear soulish realm (more blood flow to the brain) enhances fellowship with God.

Also helpful during a fast is sitting quietly in the presence of God. After praising, worshipping and ministering to Him, quiet time should be spent before God. Nothing takes the place of meditating on His Word and who He is. This shifts focus from the prevailing problems to His Magnificence. Our lives are destined to change when we spend quality time with God Almighty.

... WITH FELLOW CHRISTIANS

Our involvement in the world creates a need to enhance our relationship with our fellow man. Stress can cause people to develop bad attitudes towards each other. Sometimes these attitudes can be traced to feeling ill because of the accumulation of toxins in the body. An unclean system saps the body of the energy needed to love and express care for other people. When we have conflicts with people without a cause, there may be a need to fast. By its cleansing power, fasting unclogs the body and releases the energy needed for work, caring for the family and loving one's spouse. When fasting is accompanied by prayer and focusing on God, we are able to see our areas of weakness and where we need to improve our relationship with those who are close to us.

I remember fasting to break the habit of procrastination. I would always put off what I had to do for another day or two.

I remember working with a group on a project that needed all of our input. My procrastinating hindered the entire project. I began to fast and confess my problem to God and broke the power of procrastination over my life. This enhanced my relationship with fellow Christians and all those who were dependent upon me.

I was asked, if people easily became upset when fasting because of hunger. My answer was, yes if they are spending little or no time with God.

... WITH THE TRUE HARVEST

Luke 10:2: *"Therefore said He unto them, the harvest truly is great, but the labourers are few: pray ye therefore the Lord of the harvest, that He would send forth labourers into His harvest."*

Many times we do not recognize the true harvest. Jesus made the above statement as he looked out over the multitude. I believe one of the reasons the laborers are few is because they cannot recognize the harvest. In order to identify the harvest, we need to become more sensitive to the spirit of God. Since fasting enhances spiritual sensitivity it becomes easy to discern, by the Spirit, the people who need salvation. He will give us the insight to see the true harvest. When the eyes of our spirit are open, we can enhance fellowship with the harvest by bringing them into the kingdom. Many people do not see the harvest despite the statement Jesus made two thousand years ago.

There is no better way to become more sensitive than to mortify the flesh. Fasting increases mental alertness and focus.

Countless people who have fasted for lengthy periods witness to the clarity of thought and mental alertness. This state of being sharpens spiritual sensitivity, making people more in tuned with God and His will. Imagine what would happen if believers could stand together fasting and praying for lost souls. This would empower the church to break the fetters that keep people's ears deaf to the message of salvation.

The harvest is comprised of people whose appearance, smell and mannerism may be unpleasant. This is why most believers' eyes are blinded to the harvest. They are not people we would like to be identified with. Believers need to go before God and enhance fellowship with Him, which will in turn enhance our fellowship with fellow Christians and those whom the Lord has identified as the harvest. We need to petition God daily, asking Him to give us sensitivity to the harvest. A greater fellowship with the harvest can render us available to them. Jesus said, *"The harvest truly is great, but labourers are few..."* The laborers are few because many of them do not understand how to fellowship with the true harvest.

Points to Remember
• The fast-paced life we lead robs us of meaningful time of fellowship with God. **(Mark 12:30)**

• Without a conscious effort to shift focus from life's endless demands to God, the relationship with God is in jeopardy.

• Because of the amount of energy used by the digestive system, a person usually gets sluggish after a meal. Fasting utilizes the energy that would otherwise be used by digestion, applying it to the prayer, worship, praise and reaching out to God.

• Fasting shifts the focus from the prevailing circumstances to the Magnificence and Omnipotence of God.

• Stress saps the body's energy needed to love and enhance fellowship with fellow believers. Fasting unclogs the system and redirects that energy.

• When a believer fasts, he becomes more sensitive to the people who need salvation.

• Fasting increases mental alertness and focus, promoting clear thinking.

Chapter Five

WHEN MAKING AN
IMPORTANT DECISION

"And Jehosaphat feared, and set himself to seek the Lord and proclaimed a fast throughout all Judah. And Judah gathered themselves together, to ask help of the Lord: even out of all the cities of Judah they came to seek the Lord." **II Chronicles 20:3-4**

When a person has to make an important decision and there is no room for error, he needs divine assistance. The person needs to go before God, enhancing fellowship with Him, to clearly hear His voice. The consequences of making decisions without first seeking the mind of God will always be costly. Joshua and the leaders of Israel failed to consult with God and signed a treaty with the Gibeonites. On discovering that they had been deceived, they could not change their agreement because they had sworn in the name of the Lord. The Gibeonites became a snare to Israel throughout their lives **(Joshua 9:3-19)**. Seeking God will give us the answer we could never arrive at any other way.

When the disciples were faced with pressure from Herod, they sought the Lord with fasting and:

"As they ministered to the Lord, and fasted, the Holy Ghost said, Separate me Barnabas and Saul for the work I have called them." **(Acts 13:2)**

Their obedience led to a great revival. Paul and Barnabas had clear directions from God and began to walk in His perfect will..

RELOCATING

Before deciding to relocate to a different state for work or school, one needs to hear from God. When people relocate, they usually leave fellowships to which they were assigned by God. Making that decision demands an assurance that the person moving has heard from God. As the scripture says:

"Commit to the Lord whatever you do, and your plans will succeed." **(Proverbs 16:3 NIV)** (Read also the Amplified version)

Relocating means leaving an area and moving to another area with unknown principalities and powers. The devil would love to have everyone shifted to a location where the chief principality and power of that area is the demon of their greatest weakness. If it were left up to the devil, all the lustful people should move to where the principal demon of lust lives. For this reason, people tend to gravitate to certain parts of the country where they will more comfortably and effectively live their life-style. This is why it is very important that a person relocating hears from God before making the move. God knows whether you need to move and where you need to move to. The attraction to the place where the person desires to move may be a ploy from demon spirits wanting to disrupt God's plan in his life.

WHEN CHANGING JOBS

A lot of people think that changing from one job for a better paying job means being in the perfect will of God Before changing a job, even for a better paying one, a believer must make sure that God approved of the move. If a person's weakness is the opposite sex, the new job may, unknown to the job seeker, mean working in a office with attractive co-workers. It may not be God but the devil trying to curb the believer's spiritual progress and contribution into the kingdom. The devil's aim may be to sabotage the person's integrity and ultimately God's purpose for his or her life. The enemy may lead a person into a new job where he will fall into sin or even backslide. Before changing jobs, consult God.

"Trust in the Lord with all your heart; and lean not unto thine own understanding.

In all thy ways acknowledge Him, and He shall direct they paths." **(Proverbs 3:5-6)** (Also read from the Amplified)

BEFORE ENTERING INTO MARRIAGE

For a decision such as marriage, the couple probably needs a forty day fast before making a final decision to enter into marriage. This is probably the most important fast of one's life. Weddings are usually preceded by marriage counseling. The quality of counseling I have encountered over the years in most churches could have been much better. Counseling usually focuses on two aspects that the couple should have in common, whether they are truly in love and are born again believers.

It overlooks the background of both individuals to assess their socialization processes, to truly evaluate compatibility. Marriage is so important that such a decision demands that the couple fast in order to ensure that they have heard from God. Fasting puts on hold the physical attraction and also silences the emotions to enhance spiritual sensitivity.

"House and riches are the inheritance of fathers: and a prudent wife is from the Lord." **(Proverbs 19:14)**

STARTING A BUSINESS

"But thou shalt remember the Lord thy God: for it is He that giveth thee power to get wealth, that He may establish His covenant which He sware unto thy fathers, as it is this day." **(Deuteronomy 8:18)**

"Thus saith the Lord, thy Redeemer, the Holy One of Israel: I am the Lord thy God which teacheth thee to profit, which leadeth thee by the way that thou shouldst go." **(Isaiah 48:17)**

Before investing money into anything, believers should remember that they are God's stewards and money is a blessing from Him. *"The silver is mine, and the gold mine is mine, saith the Lord of hosts."* **Haggai 2:8** God expects believers to be good stewards. Read the parable of the stewards and see how God dealt with each of them **(Matthew 25:14-28).** Stewardship involves accountability before God for the future of the family. When a person invests funds to start a business, there needs to be commitment and accountability before God.

42

The person considering this business venture needs to hear from God through fasting, praying and worshipping, prior to making a decision. Poor stewardship will cost you everything, so fast and hear from God.

ADOPTING A CHILD OR CHILDREN

"For thou possessed my reins, thou hast covered me in my mother's womb.

I will praise Thee; for I am fearfully and wonderfully made: marvelous are thy works; and that my soul knoweth right well.

My substance was not hid from thee, when I was made in secret, and curiously wrought in the lowest parts of the earth.

Thine eyes was not hid from thee, yet being unperfect; and in thy book all my members were written which in continuance were fashioned.
(Psalm 139:13-16)

A person seeking to adopt a child needs to consult God. He is the only one who has known the child prior to birth Even though there are many reasons for adoption and they all seem to make the perspective parents anxious, this is not a step to overlook. A child may look innocent and attractive but may have deep seated problems that appear years later. Most problems are only identified when these children reach adolescence. At this stage they can become violent and aggressive. These children need to be adopted, but also need parents that can afford to give a lot of love. The adoptive parents need to consult God before adopting the child or children.

Problems which come with adoption are unlike rickets, a disease caused by lack of vitamins. When the vitamins are supplied, the symptoms can disappear permanently without leaving a trace. It is not the same for emotional problems and emotional damage. Sometimes emotional damage is not detectable at an early age or may have no specific manifestations. When the child begins to interact with others, it may remind him of unpleasant early childhood experiences.

Some children are placed with adoptive parents immediately after birth. Though this may sound like a safe age to assume parenthood, scientists have proved that a child in the womb is fully conscious of the parent's emotional turmoil. At this stage the child is neither able to defend himself nor to escape this emotional assault. This may leave the child with emotional problems and adoptive parents with no knowledge of this.

When Mary was pregnant with Jesus, she visited her cousin Elizabeth who was expecting John the Baptist:

"And it came to pass, that, when Elizabeth heard the salutation of Mary, the babe leaped in her womb, and Elizabeth was filled with Holy Ghost: And she spake out with a loud voice, and said, ...For, lo, as soon as the voice of thy salutation sounded in mine ears, the babe leaped in my womb for joy." **Luke 1:41,42,44.**

"Before I formed you in the womb I knew you, before you were born I set you apart; I appointed you as a prophet to the nations." **Jeremiah 1:5**

This is concrete biblical evidence that babies in utero (in the womb) are fully sensitive to their environment and to the spirit of God. They are also emotionally vulnerable. When a child has suffered emotionally, only God through loving parents, can heal the pain. Even after selecting a child or thinking about selecting one, the prospective parent needs to take that child before God praying and seeking His approval for the adoption.

WHEN LEAVING A FELLOWSHIP

It is important to consult God when a person is deciding to leave a fellowship or a ministry. Talking to the pastor is equally important. When a member has lost confidence in the ministry and its leadership, he needs to leave the ministry. Most Christians tend to talk negatively about the ministry instead of just leaving quietly. Before leaving the fellowship it is imperative that a person truly hears from God.

When faced with the question of why they joined a particular ministry, many believers have publicly testified that they joined at God's direction. The same people fail to consult God when faced with pressure and disappointment about that particular ministry or church. Some people have hastily left ministries, and after being away for a while, came back because the one they joined was worse than the one they left. Before leaving a fellowship, please consult God with fasting and prayer.

STARTING A MINISTRY

A person who believes that God has placed him in leadership position in a ministry must hear from Him.

The same goes for a person who plans to start a ministry. Starting an independent ministry can be a serious challenge. Take it from experience. When faced with lack of financial support, and positive response to the preaching, knowing that the ministry had been started at God's command brings rest and confidence. Do not worry, God pays His child support. **(Matthew 6:25-33)** Anything you conceive that is of God like. He will support.

Most believers that think they have been called into their own ministry must confirm the timing with God. Without confirmation from God they could launch out into the ministry ill-equipped. There are certain attractions to starting a ministry, like passing business cards that list spiritual endowments and abilities. In order to successfully impact upon other people's lives one needs God's help. Whether a person has heard from God or not will not decrease the demonic onslaught against the ministry. This can cause fear and discouragement. Before starting a ministry, it is better to hear from God. The best way I know to hear from Him is to fast. Fasting silences emotions and false visions of grandeur and exposes the true challenge and it's merits. Being in the habit of seeking God for direction will positively affect everything a believer engages in; from the start of a ministry and for the rest of his life.

Because of the gravity of the decision to accept a call into the ministry, I would suggest a 40-day fast. In the face of adversity one can rest with the assurance that he fasted and heard directly from God. Adversity is no threat when a person knows that he is in the will of God.

HEARING FROM GOD IN THE MIDST OF TURMOIL

"And I set my face unto the Lord God, to seek by prayer and supplications, with fasting, and sackcloth, and ashes...

Yea, while I was speaking in prayer, even the man Gabriel, whom I had see in the vision at the beginning, being caused to fly swiftly, touched me about the time of the evening oblation.

And he informed me, and talked with me, and said, `O Daniel, I am now come forth to give thee skill and understanding.'" (Daniel 9:3,21-22)

"And Cornelius said, `Four days ago I was fasting until this hour; and at the ninth hour I prayed in my house, and, behold, a man stood before me in bright clothing,

And said, `Cornelius, thy prayer is heard, and thine alms are had in remembrance in the sight of God.'"' (Acts 10:30-31)

In both instances these men wanted to hear from God in the midst of turmoil. When they fasted, God spoke to them. We can without warning, find ourselves in the midst of confusion. During such times we need to hear from God as never before.

Men who were trailblazers in several disciplines are known to have had a disciplined life of fasting. These men changed history, were great revolutionaries, and brought reformation to the church. Jesus Christ, Ezra, Nehemiah, Esther, Martin Luther, John Knox, John Wesley, to mention just a few.

People who fast regularly for long periods of time have testified that during the fast they have attained to higher levels of mental astuteness and clarity of direction.

While most people who do not practice the discipline of fasting are bound by the fear of physical suffering, those who are disciplined in this area say fasting quickens the spirit. The easiest way to hear from God is to be available to Him on a regular basis. When we humble ourselves before God with fasting and praying, hearing from Him becomes the inevitable result.

SEVERE MARITAL PROBLEMS

Problems between husbands and wives can sometimes lead to mistrust. There could be many of things going wrong with the marriage. In the midst of the marital turmoil, both spouses need to hear from God. This is the time to seek God with fasting and prayer. Many times God will direct you to seek a qualified Christian counselor. If one spouse is a Christian and the other is clearly putting the relationship at risk, the born again spouse needs Godly insight. In extreme cases, one's life could be in danger. Quietness before the Lord allows impartation of tremendous wisdom as to what is needed during this troubled time.

SEVERE FINANCIAL PROBLEMS

Marital and financial problems usually go hand in hand. When the financial resources are strained, the marriage relationship is also affected. When a person is faced with foreclosures, or the inability to pay the mortgage or car note, that is a severe challenge.

Such situations can cause a tremendous amount of stress and anxiety. When facing such problems the believer needs to hear from God. Sometimes we can confess the Word of God without listening to what He has to say. I confess the Word of God every morning, but I need the comfort of giving Him the chance to speak directly to me concerning my financial situation.

If a believer has financial problems that causes severe anxiety, he needs to hear from God. There is no better way to hear from God than fasting. While it is comforting to get a prophetic word through someone concerning finances, hearing directly from God is better. The prophetic word should only confirm what God has already spoken to you in private. When people do not fast, pray and stay before God, they do not know God. On receiving a prophetic word some people go off on a tangent and never qualify the word for timing or direction. Spending time with God, praising, worshipping, praying and just laying down before Him, enables the believer to hear from God. When the prophetic comes to us it should be something to confirm what God has already spoken.

A prophet once gave me a word while taking an offering. He had finished ministering, and was laying hands on the people as they passed their offering. When he came to me, he stopped everything and gave me a word. The word he spoke was not new to my ears. It was something that God had already confirmed in my spirit. I was not looking for a prophetic word but getting a word motivated me more. It motivated me to complete some things that God had birthed in my life.

Be diligent in seeking God so that when a prophet gives a word from God, it will be just a confirmation.

PROBLEMS WITH YOUR CHILDREN

"And all thy children shall be taught of the Lord; and great shall be the peace of thy children." (Isaiah 54:13)

This is a promise given to every parent concerning children. I have three children. At a certain age, they tend to become more difficult to deal with than when they were younger. As they approach adulthood, they begin to think independent thoughts, wanting to do as they please, and neglect parental advice. This stage makes parenthood difficult. The difficulty arises when children want to grow up quicker than the parents can appreciate.

Sometimes this can get out of hand. This stage of parent-hood can become very challenging. This is especially true for single parent families, where a single mother is trying to raise children alone. This is the time that the parent needs to hear from God. Dealing with rebellious children is a challenge, even with a mom and dad at home.

In order to meet this challenge a parent needs to hear from God. With all the stumbling blocks Satan has set in our youth's way to destroy them, such as AIDS, crack cocaine and alcohol, panic and despair are not the attitudes parents can afford when they find out their child is in trouble. An attitude of warfare is needed and clear orders from the commander in chief. Fasting reduces stress while enhancing spiritual sensitivity during these challenging years.

LIFE'S CHALLENGES

"These things I have spoken unto you, that in me ye might have peace. In the world ye shall have tribulation: but be of good cheer; I have overcome the world." John 16:33

Life's challenges are different for everyone and Christians are not immune to them. Sometimes these challenges cause much turmoil in a believers' life. These may be marital, financial, problems with children, or a host of other things. Believers may face problems in church, in their neighborhoods, with other people or agencies they do business with. Sometimes these problems can result in false accusations.

Facing the problem of false accusation is real and quite challenging. Christians in trouble always desire that God would take care of such cases overnight. Sometimes God allows His children to go through a painful preparatory process thus giving them an experience that they will need later in life. Such experiences become helpful when one has to minister to someone going through the same kind of problem. Going through the test successfully enables the person to minister to others who go through similar trials.

There can be many life challenges, especially for those who are called to be ministers, pastors and overseers. If you are in leadership you will have to go through several life challenges. Whenever a leader makes a positive impact on the lives of other people, the enemy tries to destroy him.

Life's challenges can be very trying. A believer definitely has the ability to overcome them. One way of overcoming them is to find out what God thinks about the particular challenge. Intelligent fasting is a sure way to gain Godly insight into life's challenges. God must have seen it coming long before it got there. A person needs to hear how God wants him to approach the problem. I guarantee you, He will bring about solutions that are beyond your imagination. He is able to take you safely through any situation that life brings.

Points to Remember:
• When a person has to make an important decision, he should consult God with a period of fasting.

• Joshua's failure to consult God before making a treaty with the Gibeonites, caused him to befriend people who became a snare to the Israelites all their lives. **(Joshua 9:3-19)**

• When the disciples were faced with pressure from Herod, they fasted and God led Saul and Barnabas to start a revival.

• Consult God with fasting and praying before leaving a fellowship you were assigned to by God. **(Proverbs 16:3)**

• Changing a job, even for increased wages and better working conditions, may not be a good idea without consulting God. **(Proverbs 3:5-6)**

• Fasting before getting married is mandatory. It silences the emotions and enhances spiritual sensitivity so that you can make the right choice. **(Proverbs 19:14)**

• A good steward will always seek God before investing money into a business venture. **(Haggai 2:8)**

• When adopting a child, the adoptive couple need to seek God with fasting.

• It is impossible to detect the problems that a child has encountered by the time he or she is adopted. Only God knows the trouble that some adopted children have gone through. He is the only One qualified to match the right child with the right parents for adoption.

Chapter Six

What Happens When We Fast

When God wanted to get the attention of His people, the king or the prophet would sometimes call a fast. Many of the people were caught up in idolatry, carnality, and many customs they learned from the heathen people living near them. Calling the entire nation on a fast would get everyone to focus on God. Fasting made them sensitive to the voice of God.

Daniel fasted in acknowledgment of the sins of his fathers. **Daniel 9:3-4 *"And I set my face unto the Lord God, to seek by prayer and supplications with fasting, and with sackcloth and ashes:***

And I prayed unto the Lord my God, and made my confession, and said . . . "

Nehemiah and the returned exiles also fasted and prayed to confess their sins and return to God. **(Nehemiah 9:13)** This enabled them to rid themselves of negative sinful situations. They did not get involved in their sinful state overnight. The involvement was subtle until they found themselves deeply involved in ungodly activities. This negative physical, mental and spiritual overindulgence weakened the nation.

They were submerged up to their necks in sin and bondage that they could not get out of. They had begun to worship and believe in idol gods. Idolaters usually believed that turning away from sacrificing to idols carried a death penalty. This caused the people to maintain a more reverential attitude towards idols(gods they could see), than the true God. Fasting like nothing else could quickly rally the people of God when they lapsed into sinful ways.

Jonah 3:7 addresses one of those instances where people returned to God through fasting.

"And he caused it to be proclaimed and published through Nineveh by the decree of the king and his nobles, saying, Let neither man nor beast, herd nor flock, taste anything, let them not feed nor drink water."

This is commonly known as the story of Jonah. God sent Jonah to Nineveh to prophesy the doom that would befall the city because of their sin. Jonah refused to go because he didn't think they deserved to be warned about the impending destruction. Jonah's self righteous attitude and his free will was altered drastically by God. As the story goes, Jonah was swallowed by a whale and remained in his belly for three days. The whale finally spat him up on dry land. It was then that he decided that he would go to Nineveh and preach to the the people. Arriving in Nineveh, Jonah proclaimed what was to become of the Ninevites if they did not repent. The king decreed in the entire land that no one was to eat, taste or drink anything. The whole nation went on a **complete fast** as an expression of their **repentance**, and also to **clearly hear** from God. This fast averted God's judgment.

Sometimes rulers would decree a fast which included every person and domesticated beast. This directed the entire nation's focus on God so that His will could be carried out in the land. **(II Chronicles 20; Ezra 8:22)**

It is for a similar cause that pastors and overseers will sometimes proclaim fasts for entire congregations. Such fasts become necessary to cleanse the church of worldliness, and to refocus on God. When God reveals to the pastor that corporate sin is in the congregation, he may call a fast. Sometimes a fast is called even when the church operations may be going smoothly. It may be to avoid problems in the future, because only God knows what the church will face in the months to come. Coming before God and penitently seeking His face gives the people a chance to judge themselves and avert His judgment. God may reveal things to them personally, so that they can straighten up their act. Corporate fasts may avert embarassment and destroyed lives by stopping sin before it is exposed.

Matthew 17:14-21 is a controversial scripture. Many people feel this scripture should not be in the Bible. Some Bible translations like the Holman's New International Version have this scripture removed from the text and italicized as a footnote at the bottom of the page. They make the reader forget its existence. This verse belongs to the text and we really need to accept it, especially in the light of the power that comes through fasting.

Matthew 17:21: *"Howbeit this kind goeth not out but by prayer and fasting."* Jesus spoke these words after His disciples had failed to cast a demon out of a boy. After Jesus delivered the boy from demonic oppression, the disciples asked Him why they had failed.

Jesus first remarked, *"Because of your unbelief. Howbeit, this kind goeth not out but by prayer and fasting."* Most theologians do not even want to mention the last part of this scripture. It cannot be left out, we just have to embrace it and believe what it says is important.

Fasting should always be accompanied by prayer, worship and praise. In this verse, Jesus makes a statement concerning the work of the Holy Spirit. It is the Holy Spirit who gives the power to cast out any kind of demon. This also puts emphasis on the confidence and faith in God needed by a person through whom the Holy Spirit works. When He tells His disciples that, *"Howbeit this kind goeth not out but by prayer and fasting"* He refers to the work of the Holy Spirit and their faith and confidence in God. I believe that they go together. It was because of their unbelief that they could not cast out the demon. Spending quality time in prayer with fasting will always enhance your relationship with God because he can speak to you. And we know that faith cometh by hearing the words of God. Because prayer and fasting is always accompanied by praise, worship, and reading the word of God it will always increase our faith.

Jesus made another statement in **Matthew 9:19-20** about fasting. The Pharisees complained that they fasted all the time, but His disciples did not fast. Jesus responded:

"Can the children of the bride chamber mourn, as long as the bridegroom is with them? But the days will come when the bridegroom shall be taken from them, and then shall they fast." This implied that when Jesus left, the disciples should and would be fasting and praying regularly.

They could not cast the demon out because they did not fast. It had nothing to do with the power of the Holy Spirit. The Holy Spirit is always willing and able to do what He has to do. Just like Jesus had suggested, the problem was their faith. Maybe they needed to get closer to God in order to better understand Him, before casting out those types of demons.

According to **Matthew 17:21**, prayer and fasting prepare Christians for the **work of ministry**. Ministering to God with praise, worship and prayer during a fast makes believers more sensitive to His voice, while sharpening their overall spiritual sensitivity. Sensitivity to the spirit of God enhances the believer's ability to understand God's Word and thus His Will. The increased ability to hear the voice of God through fasting allows God to reveal Himself. This creates a closeness to God, and an assurance of His commitment to His Word, which when heard(understood), increases faith.

Romans 10:17: *"So then faith cometh by hearing, and hearing by the word of God."* By the same token, fasting makes us more sensitive to what we hear and read about God. Prayer, praise and worship enable us to have fellowship with God, in whom we have the utmost confidence. With this deeper sensitivity and enlightened fellowship with God, we can carry out with confidence the perfect will of God. This highlights the significance of prayer and fasting.

Prayer and fasting does not make God do what he is unwilling to do. Neither does it make the Spirit work any stronger or any better. It does something to us. Whatever God does during this dispensation, He does it through man.

Heaven moves when earth bids. Prayer and fasting make us better vessels for the Spirit of God to work through.

Psalm 35:1-18 (13): *"But as for me, when they were sick, my clothing was sackcloth: I humbled my soul with fasting; and my prayer returned into mine own bosom."*

In this scripture, David bemoans the attitude of the people who had wronged him. He declares that when his enemies were sick, he prayed for them. He went to God and ministered to Him, humbling his soul with fasting, rendering himself more sensitive to hear God's voice. Persecution by others brings about a natural negative reaction towards the perpetrator. If we follow David's example, fasting and ministering to God with prayer, praise and worship proves to be the most effective way of dealing with adversity. Holding your peace and allowing Him to advise and comfort us as we safely sail through the adversity.

At the same time, He can deal with your persecutors any way He chooses. While the natural man clubs the culprit out of frustration, ministering to God brings about healing. David was bent on doing right, no matter what his enemies did to him. When they were sick or had any need, David prayed for them. Sometimes when facing persecution, the best posture is to be quiet, stop eating, and get more sensitive to God while he takes care of the situation. This attitude towards persecutors guarantees that God will take care of the situation. Before you know it, He will get the situation taken care of.. Receive God's comfort and advice while He deals with your persecutors.

Remember, He can deal with them any way He wants to, and more effectively than anyone. When He has dealt with them, they will no longer bother you.

FASTING ETIQUETTE

Matthew 6:16-18. *"Moreover when ye fast, be not as the hypocrites, of sad countenance: for they disfigure their faces, that they may appear unto men to fast. Verily I say unto you, They have their reward.*

But thou, when thou fastest; anoint thy head, and wash thy face;

That thou appear not unto men to fast, but unto thy Father, which seeth in secret: and thy Father which seeth in secret, shall reward thee openly."

It is important to understand that fasting is very personal and is between the person concerned and God. Do not fast to impress other people. That is forbidden in Scripture. While on a fast, some people look for approval because of the hunger suffered. They go around looking pitiful and hungry, drawing attention to themselves. They may be doing this to impress others about their spiritual fortitude. This attitude does not impress God at all. It does inform others how much you fast, exalting you in man's eyes. Fasting is essentially an expression of deepest humility by man towards God. It has nothing to do with your neighbors and friends. If it is done to impress others by appearing to suffer, it becomes vanity.

Some people perceive fasting as tough to the physical body.

While fasting may seem to weaken the body, it is in essence, cleansing the body and strengthening the spirit man. No matter how long the fast, no one should discern that you are fasting by merely observing your appearance. I am not saying that there is anything wrong with telling people that you are on a fast. There should be a reason for telling others that you are fasting. This will help eliminate unnecessary involvement in certain unfruitful activities and foolish conversation. When people offer you something to eat, it becomes necessary to tell them that you are on a fast. There is nothing wrong with telling your family that you are on a fast. But if you are telling them just to impress them, that is wrong. Fasting is between you and God. God knows what you want to accomplish by fasting, and He will reward you personally for it.

As the Scripture declares that God will reward you openly for what you have accomplished in private. No one will know what you have accomplished in fasting until after you have fasted and they begin to see the fruit and the changes in your life.

Just because some one goes on a fast does not mean that they are going to receive tremendous benefits. Many uninformed people have fasted and did not reap much in terms of spiritual benefits. Instead they have harmed their physical bodies by abstaining from food and drink for many days. This type of fasting leaves a person in such a miserable state that what they would have gained spiritually is negated by the fact that they did so poorly physically and emotionally. Chapter Eight will give insight on the do's and don'ts of fasting.

Points to Remember

• Fasting made God's people sensitive to God's instruction. Daniel fasted to acknowledge the sins of his fathers, after which God sent an angel to bring his reply **(Daniel 9:3-4)**. So did Nehemiah and the returned exiles **(Nehemiah 9:1-3)**.

• Jonah preached and the convicted Ninevites returned to God through fasting and acknowledgments of their sin, thus averting God's judgement **(Jonah 3:7)**

• People fasted when they faced an unavoidable attack from the enemy. **(II Chronicles 20; Ezra 8:22)**

• Prayer and fasting gives the believer confidence that the power of God will work in his life to drive out demons. **(Matthew 17:14-21)**

• Just as faith comes by hearing the Word of God, fasting makes a believer more sensitive to what he hears and reads about God.

• Ministering to God by fasting, with prayer, praise and eating the Word proves to be the best and most effective way to deal with your adversaries. **(Psalm 35:13)**

• A person fasting should not attract attention to himself. When a person fasts in secret, the Lord will reward him openly.
(Matthew 6:16-18)

Chapter Seven

Fasting the Soul

Most writings concerning fasting have emphasized either the spiritual or physical benefits but not the emotional benefits of fasting. Triune man must benefit from fasting in all three aspects of his being. The soulish part of man is the keeper and dispenser of the emotions, feelings and thought processes of the intellect. There are only three ways the soulish part of man's nature can be effected:

• Stimuli that come through the five senses. This can also be termed experiences.

• Stimuli that come from stored memories, in other words, from the conscious and subconscious memory bank.

• Stimuli that come from the adversary, the devil.

Now we understand that the devil has access to our mental capacity. He can plant thoughts into our minds. He cannot make us entertain any thoughts, but he has the ability to place a thought in our minds. The thoughts he usually plants in our minds go hand in hand with our experiences and what comes into our conscious minds from our memory. For instance, if you are watching a television program and see an attractive member of the opposite sex, the devil can plant a lustful, unholy thought in your mind.

The Bible says that the thoughts of the righteous are right **Proverbs 12:5.** Many negative thoughts that a wholesome Christian may have do not come from their own heart and spirit, they are planted by the enemy.

All three types of stimuli affecting the soulish part of man work in conjunction with one another. What we experience by way of our sensory perception precipitates what is released from our stored memory. Likewise, it is often what dictates which thoughts will be planted by the enemy in our minds. When we go to a certain place that we think we have been before, the memories from our memory bank come into our conscious minds as we experience the surroundings, trying to remember.

I remember meeting someone that I had not seen for years. We looked at each other, trying to remember where we knew each other from. We had to rely on our memory bank and our conversation to refresh ourselves. A lot of other thoughts sprang up before the right one surfaced. Sometimes we have to help the memory bank along. I inquired where I knew him from, and he replied, "Maybe from school. What school did you attend?" "Wayne State." "Well, I went to Wayne State, too." This is how the memory bank begins to bring up past experiences until you can communicate to find out where you know the person from. The experiences, or those outward stimuli that we get from our senses, precipitate what comes out of our memory bank.

The same thing happens when you see an attractive person of the opposite sex. This stimuli may precipitate a memory of someone similar that you had been attracted to. When the memory bank brings it up, the devil can come and plant an unwholesome thought in your mind at that instant.

Although the enemy can plant a negative thought, we do not have to entertain it. **Philippians 4:8 ...** *"think on these things."*

Now that we understand about how our experiences are related to our thought process, we can explore how fasting can help us emotionally.

In **Ephesians 6**, Paul charges the church at Ephesus to understand that there is definitely a hidden opposition that influences human beings.

"For we wrestle not against flesh and blood but against principalities, against powers, against the rulers of the darkness of this world, against spiritual wickedness in high places." **Ephesians 6:12**

Paul was writing to born-again believers in Jesus Christ. Most of what Paul wrote in the New Testament was written to Christians. True born-again Christians cannot be demon possessed, but demonic influence and oppression is alive and well in the body of Christ.

Many Christians are being demonically influenced. Taking it to the extremes, one can say that all Christians are demonically influenced, in varying degrees. Everyone has been assigned cohorts of the devil to influence him in a negative way. Just like Jesus sent to us the Holy Spirit to lead, guide and help us live the life of Christ, there are demons assigned to all of us to deceive and force us into a life of sin. To understand how fasting can truly benefit us emotionally, we must first see how emotional problems begin and are maintained.

Depression is by far the most common emotional disorder among Christians. A long time ago depression was believed to be for non-Christians only, but now we know better. Let us take a look at our model of soulish influence to see how this disease is perpetuated. Depression is an emotional disorder that develops over time in response to stimuli (experiences) and thought processes. It is aimed at ultimately destroying our importance or self-worth. This is how this works: At a very young age we are told that we are stupid or dumb because we could not give the right answer to what we were told was a very simple question. It may have taken us too long to put together a puzzle which made others refer to us as not so bright, or dumb. When someone you love, or respect, or both, tells you things about yourself, you believe them. If a parent or someone important to you told you that you were dumb, you would eventually believe them. As time goes on this belief about yourself is reinforced by parents, teachers, peers and many of your own experiences.

The process continues with each negative experience. In time you build a huge reservoir of negative memories. These memories of previous failures surface from the subconscious memory bank in response to negative stimuli to support this negative belief. Finally, thoughts planted by the devil (at that instant) in response to the same negative stimuli, also support this negative belief. This process repeated over and over as you grow, affects your behavior and attitude. It also destroys self confidence by instilling a belief that you are not intelligent at all. If you feel that you are not intelligent, then your worth is diminished, and eventually you feel worthless. This is by far one of the major causes of depression.

This is just one example, but there are many others, each one as diverse as the experiences we have. Whether it be that you are labeled dumb, ugly, clumsy, fat, weird, or you were neglected, which makes you feel less important, you could end up suffering from depression.

There are many new medications that treat depression quite well. Most people who suffer from depression may take these medications on and off for years.

How Fasting Helps Us Emotionally

When we begin fasting, we deprive our bodies of nourishment at the same time making our spirit and soul more sensitive to God. Just like fasting from food, one needs to fast from things that constantly bombard the soul (emotions, mind, intellect).

I recommend a triune fast. This means fasting to benefit spirit, soul and body. Triune fasting is abstinence from food, abstinence from all of the stimuli that bombard the soul (TV, radio, newspaper, magazines), and abstinence from a lack of communion with God. A person can fast to rest the emotions, just like you give your body rest when you fast from food and unnecessary activities. Many times people who are fasting have to work with disturbing individuals. These people always talk negatively, and speak about the worst things in life. Being around such people does not exhort you or make you feel better. When fasting, you should avoid such people. In order to benefit emotionally from a fast avoid watching movies. Christians should avoid movies which evoke negative emotions(fear, sexual, rebellion, the unknown). Scary and suspenseful movies are not beneficial while fasting. This emotional baggage should be avoided.

When people are fasting physically, they should also be fasting emotionally.Fasting the soulish realm from all of the emotional garbage and feeding the soul and Spirit the Word of God, is a time of refreshing. Whenever you feed your soul with the Word, and deprive it of all negative emotions, a tremendous change takes place. This enhances clarity of thought and you truly begin to understand God's Word. When you read or listen to the Word of God repeatedly, God speaks to you. Sometimes after reading several scriptures, one seems to jump out at you. That is the scripture God is drawing your attention to in order to speak to you. After fasting the soulish realm from all of the garbage, you have clarity of thought when you read or listen to God's Word. You get so much more out of the Word because it becomes much more alive.

The Word of God says, *"My sheep hear my voice"* **John 10:27a**. There will be no question about the voice of God that you hear. When you are fasting, you will receive great revelation from reading and listening to the Word of God. When God speaks, you will identify His voice without a doubt. You will attain to such clarity of mind that if the devil speaks to you (as he sometimes will), you will recognize his voice immediately

During the 22nd day of my first 40-day fast, the Lord began to speak to me. The same day the devil also spoke to me. There are many times prior to fasting when I heard what I thought was the voice of God in my spirit. I would wonder whether that was God, the devil or me. During my soulish fast, there was absolutely no doubt whose voice was speaking to me.

I could clearly distinguish and immediately discern between my thoughts, God's voice, or the voice of the enemy. I could discern God's voice because I was fasting from the emotional baggage that I carried every day. When fasting from all of the emotional garbage, the soulish realm gets an opportunity to rest. I long now to be there again. I will fast more and more often because I long to be in that state where there is no doubt in my mind when God speaks.

The Bible says, *"My sheep hear my voice, and I know them, and they follow me."* **John 10:27** *"And a stranger will they not follow, but will flee from him: for they know not the voice of strangers."* **John 10:5**. Good and constant communication between a shepherd and his sheep promotes familiarity. The sheep will eventually know the shepherd's voice. Thus, we also will know God's voice when we spend quality time with Him, while fasting our soulish realm.

We talked about depression and how it is perpetuated. Fasting the soulish realm also gives some relief to those who suffer from depression. Fasting has to be accompanied by feeding on the Word of God by listening to the Bible on tape or reading it, watching Christian television programs, and meditating(on God's Word). Positive experiences with less or no contact with negative experiences uplifts the spirit man. When your experiences are positive, they trigger good and decent memories. The evil thoughts will be so clearly discernible that it will never be entertained by your mind. Any diabolic thought opposed to the joy and the peace that you experience from your emotional fast will be dismissed without much effort. This will stop the process of depression.

When a child of God listens to His Word with a clear mind and positive experiences, he is able to grasp the truth about new birth and being a new creature in Christ. The old man and his depressing experiences has passed away and everything has become new, you are seated with christ in the heavenly places. When a person listens to the Word of God over and over during soulish fasting, the devil does not have any negative thoughts to plant. Memories are prompted by experiences that come in. Positive thoughts spawn positive memories, making it easy to remember what God has done. You will remember how God provided for you when you had nothing to eat. An encumbered soul makes it easy to tap into the strength of the inner man when faced with any trouble. When the devil plants anything in your mind, you immediately discard it. During a soulish fast, you stop that process of experiences deposited into your soul, and you begin to reclaim your mental and spiritual strength. This can only be possible when you starve yourself of those things that tax your emotions in a negative way.

Points to Remember

• The three stimuli that affect the soulish part of man are the five senses, stored memories, and stimuli that come from the devil.

• These stimuli work hand in hand, making our minds susceptible to Satanic attacks. **Ephesians 6:12**

• Although Christians cannot be demon possessed, they can be oppressed and influenced by demons.

• Depression is the most common disorder associated with demonic oppression among Christians.

• When a believer fasts the soulish realm, his mind is released from the weights and cares of this world to be able to hear from God. **John 10:5**

• Fasting the soulish realm accompanied by prayer, listening to God, and studying the written word, enhances clarity of thought.

• A person who is fasting should try to avoid unnecessary contact with disturbing individuals.

Chapter Eight

Some Important Facts About Fasting

This section will deal with:
- How to fast
- The length of time of a fast
- Your reason for fasting

A person should fast on a regular basis and the fast should not be for less than twenty-four hours. Fasting for part of the day, even for many days, is of little benefit. A modified fast *(see Chapter Nine)*, is where you eat very small amounts of fruits, vegetables, and grains so the appetite is never satisfied. For those who are new to fasting, I suggest a twenty-four hour fast each week for several weeks to get used to controlling your hunger. Then progress to a three day fast each month, and then move on to a seven -day fast every three months. Before long you will be able to handle at least one long fast (twenty-one, thirty, or forty days) annually. I also suggest that three-fourths of any fast longer than a day be a modified fast and the remaining fourth be liquids only. Never fast without water. You will benefit physically, mentally and spiritually from following these fasting guidelines.

As a rule, the more severe the problem, the longer one should endeavor to fast. In more challenging situations one may need to stay before God longer in order to hear from Him. The regularity of the fasts depends upon the person's priority and urgency of need.

The length of a fast should be determined before beginning the fast. Do not start a fast hoping to go as long as you can. It is only wise to determine the length of the fast before you start. Fasting for long periods of time can hurt you if you don't have a clear understanding of exactly what to do while on the fast. In chapters 4 and 5, we discussed the major reasons for fasting. The reason for fasting should be determined before starting your fast also. It can be as specific as wanting to hear from God before making a decision about marriage or as general as just wanting to renew the intimate fellowship you once shared with God. It should be determined prior to starting because it will direct your prayer and scripture selection.

When you finally begin to fast, try to find days that you can spend time alone. If you are married or live with others this may be difficult. During your fast, try not to talk as much, unless of course you are sharing Christ. If you feel you must fast for a short time, try to find some one to fast with you. Groups of people can fast for short periods such as choirs, deacons, prayer groups, or department heads. Please notify your pastor prior to any fast so there is no conflict with important events. If multiple short fast are done regularly, longer fast may not be needed.

People who fast on a regular basis reduce the challenges of life. Since fasting enhances our relationship with God, people who fast on a regular basis have less trouble with "besetting sin and the weights" problems. The weights I am referring to are the cares of life that so easily beset us. I believe that we would not have as many problems if we constantly kept our temples clean.

Failure to cleanse the temple regularly clutters the temple, which opens the door to physical and emotional attacks that keep us bound.

HEALTH CONCERNS

Food depravation can be dangerous, especially if a person is taking medications. People on any kind of medication, suffering from any chronic diseases like diabetes or lupus should consult a doctor before fasting for any length of time. When people with chronic illness fast to keep the temple clean, their health conditions improve. People who suffer from chronic illness can follow a fasting program without depriving themselves of nutrition. Multiple supplements can be taken during a fast to aid in proper nutrition. A practical reference to vitamins, minerals, herbs, and food supplements can be purchased at any health food store. Your doctor should be consulted before fasting or taking supplements.

PERSONAL DECISION

Fasting has to be voluntary and personal. A person who does not want to go on a fast should not be forced to do so. If a person feels inconvenienced by fasting at a particular time, he should not fast. Fasting without conviction could leave a person in a worse condition because they did not fast the proper way. It would make such a person vulnerable and possibly rob him of the benefits of fasting. There are some pastors that force members to fast by threatening them. Using fear is a form of witchcraft and is used to control members of the church. Fasts that are forced on others will cause them problems.

ENTERTAINMENT

Fasting increases our sensitivity to the spirit world. Not only the spirit of God, but demonic spirits as well. We should be careful of exposure to the secular media such as television, movies, books, magazines and radio. The media is filled with several ungodly opportunities for our minds and what we think about can eventually find itself affecting our spirit. This is why it is important to avoid watching ungodly programs. There may be nothing wrong with Christian TV, especially preaching and praise music programs. These programs feed the spirit, giving strength during the fast. Watching anything else contaminates the soul and weakens the will to fast. The same goes for newspapers and books. Fasting leaves the body weak, and the soul and spirit vulnerable. Be careful what you expose yourself to during the fast.

MARRIAGE

"Defraud ye not one the other, except it be with consent for a time, that ye may give yourselves to fasting and prayer, and come together again, that Satan tempt ye not for your incontinency." **I Corinthians 7:5**

Husbands and wives should abstain from any sexually pleasurable activity. Many people think that fasting means only sexual abstinence, but will kiss, hug and pamper one another. There is nothing wrong with a hug, but you should not get any physical enjoyment out of each other during the time of your fasting. Fasting is setting oneself apart for God, not for his or her spouse.

76

A person exposes himself to a lot of different spirits when he expresses himself sexually. There may be nothing wrong with sharing the same bed, hugging and coming in contact with each other. But it should not be done for pleasure during a fast.

DATING

People who are dating should abstain from physical contact all together. There may be nothing wrong with chatting on the phone or telling each other good night, but please avoid physical contact. The enemy would like to have you go too far so he can torment you with guilt.

WORK

Since fasting renders people more sensitive emotionally, arguments and confrontations may easily erupt. These should be avoided. This is why I recommend staying away from work, if possible, while fasting. Sometimes stress related to work can bring about confrontations and arguments. Arguing should be totally avoided during the fast. Most people cannot stay away from work while fasting, but they can avoid confrontations.

THE WORD

There should be a constant exposure to the Word of God. Constant means throughout the entire fast. This means every minute of every day, when possible. For some people, this might be impossible, but strive to make exposure to the word of God as constant as humanly possible. This may be through reading the Bible, listening to sermon and music tapes, or the Bible on tape.

An excellent form of this exposure to the word while fasting can be done by playing the word on an auto reverse tape player while sleeping. One time while I was fasting, I had a group of believers pray together in my office while I taped them. When I arrived home, I played the tape and was blessed by the prayers of the saints. The same anointing that was in the office was transferred to my home. I cannot stress how important that was. Listening to prayer is invaluable during a fast. It strengthens the will power to pray while fasting. When hunger pangs come, they are a remainder of man's dependence on God as the ultimate life giving source. Do not take hunger pangs as an attack, but an alarm clock declaring that it is time to call on God. One may find personal preaching tapes helpful during this time. I do not suggest that you expose yourself to preachers unless you agree with the preaching.

CONCLUDING A FAST

The final days or day should be spent in seclusion with worship, praise, meditation, and being quiet before the Lord. Though there may be stumbling blocks that make it impossible to be secluded, do not allow anything to stop you from fasting. During a forty day fast it may be impossible to seclude yourself for the last ten days, but do it for as many days as you can. A person can gain a lot by being alone with God during this time. Avoid the telephone or talking to anybody and be available only to God.

Water should be the first thing consumed after a fast, and a gradual introduction to solid foods, similar to the way food was depleted during the fast. For the first 7 to 10 days, especially after an extended fast, meat should be avoided. It will probably make you sick because the body has been deprived of it for some time.

Since the body has not had to digest meats and processed foods during the fast, reintroduction of complex foods should be gradual. Solid food should be introduced the same way it was depleted. A person can consider starting with fish and chicken, and then working up to heavier meat, like lamb and beef. It may take up to 2 weeks before the body gets used to meat. These are some important tips about fasting. Observing these tips will save a person many problems. It will make the fast more effective and easier to accomplish the ultimate goal for fasting and that is to communicate with God. Anyone who does not know how to hear from God needs to fast.

THINGS NOT TO BE CONSUMED DURING ANY FAST:

Coffee or tea except herbal teas with honey. Do not consume any stimulants during any fast.

Candy, chips, cake, pies or any kind of junk food: These have empty calories and are filled with non-foods that may encourage toxic build up in the system.

Gum: Chewing gum stimulates the flow of digestive juices, which may cause a stomach discomfort. When the stomach is empty, the flow of gastric juices should not be encouraged.

White granulated sugar: This causes fermentation of food in the stomach and may encourage toxic build up. It should not be consumed during a fast.

No meat, fish or any kind of seafood during your fast.

There should be **no smoking or tobacco use.**

Eggs or dairy products should not be consumed.

THINGS TO AVOID DURING A FAST:

Secular television or radio, secular newspaper or magazines.

No sports events, theater, concerts and secular videos at all. Some Christian videos are good if they are not entertainment videos. A lot of Christian videos have more entertainment in them than the word of God. Abstinence from secular entertainment during a fast helps the soul to fast too. This brings about emotional rest and restoration of the soul. If the time slots usually taken to watch secular television programs and reading the paper were devoted strictly to listening and talking to God, much could be gained from a fast.

THINGS TO DO DURING EVERY FAST:

Drink water: Steamed-distilled water, six to eight glasses daily.

Spirulina: These are tablets which are whole food products. They are available at any health food store. Take three to five of them in the morning and afternoon. Because you will not be eating meat or any protein, the spirulina has all the protein needed. Anybody going on a fast for more than three days should be on spirulina. I take alfalfa, a similar herb, on a daily basis, whether I am on a fast or not.

Drink only organic fruit or vegetable juices (available at health food stores). Freshly squeezed juices from organic fruit and vegetables are even more beneficial.

If you are fasting for long periods you should consider a cleansing enema every four to seven days.

The enema is optional for a fast seven days or less.

Take **a colon cleansing fiber** tablet or powder with water daily. I suggest a colon cleansing fiber with acidophilus or the kind of bacteria that would put the normal flora back into the colon.

Herb teas: Four to five cups a day. Drinking herbal teas can be a substitute for water.

There are different herb teas: pau d' arco, echinacea, rose hips tea, red clover tea, alfalfa tea and chamomile tea to mention just a few. There are even detoxifying teas that are excellent during a fast.

A person on medication should **consult a doctor before going on a fast.**

Do mild exercises.

During a fast a person can do arm rolls and stretching exercises for ten minutes a day. This is safe.

For a person on a long fast, oatmeal, malt-o-meal or any of those cereals can substitute for each other. A meal may not consist of more than a small bowl of cereal. A person that is fasting should not be eating to fill up, but is eating to sustain the body. The cereal can be sweetened with one teaspoon of honey or brown sugar. Remember that these are concentrated food stuffs with a lot of natural sugar. Wheat toast, a bagel, or raisin English muffin can be eaten with the cereals.

Brown rice, can substitute for the vegetable salad. .

Kyo green, green magma, spirulina or alfalfa tablets can substitute for each other. Organic fresh fruit can be substituted with dry un-sulfured fruit. There are other nutrients that are optional. Some people take them every day. I take vitamins and minerals, antioxidants and enzymes daily.

Points to Remember

• When a person fasts, he should at least fast for twenty-four hours. Fasting for less than a day at a time is of little benefit.

• The length of the fast should be determined before beginning the fast.

• For those who want to fast regularly, one day a week or three days a month is sufficient.

• Two-thirds of any fast longer than a day should be a modified fast.

• People who fast on a regular basis reduce the risk of being overweight.

• Fasting rests the vital organs and rids the body of toxins.

• Mentally you will avoid thoughts and confrontations that bring about stress.

• Spiritually you will become more sensitive to the will of God concerning your life. You will learn to trust Him, no matter what life presents to you.

• No matter how long you fast, you only fast one day at a time.

Chapter Nine

Fasting the Link to the Seventh Day

The Spirit of the Lord compelled me to fast to ease the pain that I was feeling. I had recently begun to go through the toughest time of my life. My fast would be 40 days. It would be a modified fast, eating only things that grew from the earth, and very little. I wondered why God wanted my fast to be so long. What was wrong with a 10 day fast or a 20 day fast. God had spoken clearly and only after my fast did I understand the significance of the number 40.

It was the most wonderful time in my life. The pain that I was feeling seemed to be suspended. The circumstances of the pain were the same, but the pain was not there. God began to talk to me concerning the earlier part of my life and many of the things that I had experienced He began to show me that some of the choices I made were good, but were not in His will for my life. Day after day during my fast became a time of learning about God and more about myself. About halfway through the fast, the Spirit of God began to speak to me and I began to give birth to songs, revelations concerning the Word, special words for individuals and thoughts to share with the Body of Christ. God revealed to me the origin of certain of my desires that were not holy and gave me complete deliverance from them. The Lord told me that my work for Him would change and that my sacrifice would be greater, but His work through my life would be greater.

There would be a time of purging and then a time of preparation for a greater work by the Holy Spirit. During my fast and time of my studies, I came upon a grave secret concerning the Devil. Satan cannot wage battles for long periods of time, and 40 days of prayer and fasting can surely weaken and almost always completely break his power.

Forty is a very significant number when we wage war in the spirit. Time of warfare of 40 days or more will almost always defeat the enemy, so my fast had to be 40 days to be most effective. If we look to the Word of God, we see that Moses lived his life in three sets of 40 years. He was 40 years old when he left the affluent life in Egypt, he was 80 years old when God called him in the desert through the burning bush, and he was 120 years old when he died after viewing the promised land. When God wanted to give his people a new revelation, Moses remained on the mountain for 40 days. When God wanted to completely destroy sinful men on earth, the rain came 40 days and 40 nights. The period of time it takes for a human being to conceive and give birth is 40 weeks. Forty days of fasting and prayer gives us the strength to give birth to the things God has placed in our spirit. The number 40 is also the number of testing. Jesus was encouraged (the Bible says driven) into the wilderness by the Holy Spirit for forty days of fasting, testing, and preparation for the work He had to do. So we can completely destroy habits of sin and cleanse our lives through fasting. The number 40 was significant when God judged wickedness in leadership. Jonah finally went to Nineveh. He preached to the nation for 40 days. They listened and their destruction was averted when their leader ordered everyone to fast.

David defeated Goliath and thus the army of the Philistines after Goliath terrorized the army of Israel for 40 days. The Spirit of the Lord began to speak to me concerning the last days. In **Peter II 3:8** it states that *"one day is with the Lord is as a thousand years, and a thousand years as one day."*

As we approach the new millennium, we enter into an important time, the seventh day. The year 2000 marks the beginning of the seventh day of grace. From Adam to Christ was 4,000 years or four days, from Christ to now has been 2,000 years or two days, and from the year 2000 to 3000 is the seventh day. We will witness during this time unparalleled manifestations by the Spirit of God through man. We have seen glimpses of this throughout the sixth day. People are being healed, delivered and the Word going forth to encourage and change lives. But these manifestations are nothing like what we will see in the seventh day.

There are four major attributes that have come back into the church, and it is no mistake that the last movement has reentered the church just before the seventh day. The four major attributes first existed in the early church and was instrumental in the rapid growth and tremendous courage exhibited by the Christians. The strength of the church was in its leaders ability to understand and walk in these attributes, led by the Holy Spirit.

The major attributes the Apostles moved in were: justification, holiness, faith and authority. The Apostles had an unwavering understanding that the finished work of Christ was what justified their salvation. Most early church leaders were eyewitnesses of his death and resurrection.

They also understood that although they received salvation, the outward show of Holy living was their greatest witness. God required them to live Holy then and he requires a Holy life from us now. A Holy life is impossible for anyone to live by his own strength, but faith in the accomplishment of our Lord and King gives us the ability to strive toward a Holy life. Faith was not in short supply because the early leaders witnessed Jesus so many times operate in faith and was always quick to recognize many who also operated in faith. The fourth attribute all the early leaders walked in was authority. These leaders knew who they were in Christ and had a boldness, almost cocky attitude about their authority in the face of the enemy. These attributes complimented one another and we saw the tremendous effect they had in the early church.

Satan began to infiltrate the church with philosophies and doctrines that had little or no real truth and caused divisions concerning the validity of these attributes. Satan also began to kill the leaders one by one. Before long people believed that justification was not only because of the finished work of Christ, but attendance to church, adherence to rules, hours of praying and circumcision. Holiness became something you did instead of something you were. Faith in God was for his providence in your life because all those to be chosen were already chosen. Faith really became hope that you would be chosen, and after being chosen then hope that you could do enough to get into heaven.

Authority was not spoken of and certainly if anyone had authority it was the highest of leadership.

People believed that no ordinary Christian could move in the gifts of the spirit and the Apostles were dead, so there was no authority in the church. The church became controlled by the governing authority and for centuries operated without these four major attributes. The Holy Spirit began to speak to Martin Luther who, against great Demonic opposition began to restore the doctrine of justification into the church. Martin Luther proved with the Word of God that justification for our salvation was due to the finished work of Jesus Christ, and not in works.

Next, the Holy Spirit began to speak to Charles Parham and William Seymour and from a small church on Azusa Street in California, the doctrine of the Holiness by the indwelling of the Holy Spirit is restored into the church. The Holy Spirit then speaks to a Baptist boy named Kenneth Hagin, who accepts Christ as his Savior and is healed of an incurable disease. He would go on through the teachings of E.W. Kenyon and others, to teach the Body of Christ the importance of faith, bringing the third attribute back into the Body of Christ.

The Holy Spirit then speaks to a down-to-earth, common man by the name of Bill Hammon, who against Demonic opposition, began to teach the importance of the five fold ministry gifts operating in the church. He taught that the five fold ministry gifts were to "perfect" the Body of Christ and that the Body of Christ could do the work of the ministry. He was instrumental in bringing back into the church the fourth and final attribute of authority. By concentrating on the prophetic and apostolic, he has given the church the authority for the seventh day.

As with every attribute in the church some people get off on a tangent, taking one attribute while lacking the other. They have Holiness without faith, or faith without Holiness or authority without Holiness. A seventh day man of God must have a clear understanding and embrace them all. In the sixth day we have seen manifestations of the Spirit of God through man. We have witnessed it in meetings, in prophetic gatherings, in great faith teachers meetings, and some of the great healing meetings. All of this has only been the tip of the iceberg in comparison with the manifestations of the Spirit we are about to see. It is no mistake that the last two attributes to be restored to the body has come just before the seventh day.

It is also no mistake that the resurgence of fasting has come on the threshold of the new millennium. Most people in the body have been fasting only once in a while to get closer to God after drifting away. Even when fasting regularly, like weekly, it is of little importance, because it is usually less than twenty-four hours and is primarily a fast from food. We have recently begun to see fasting take on new meaning for many in the body. Now, even some well known leaders are beginning to fast seriously and intelligently. Fasting has become something that is done regularly to God, for the body of Christ.

In day six God works through man, and man gets most of the glory. We say it is God, but people attend meetings because of personalities. The Spirit manifests through men of God the minimum of what the Spirit could actually do. Most of the crowd that comes to conferences are in unbelief, bothered by the cares of life.

There is such a tremendous spirit of misunderstanding brewing that the enemy can easily confuse many Christians searching for something better in God. People spend large sums of money to come to conferences and get very little that is truly life changing. Our conferences become an occasion to patronize non-Christian restaurants, because we love to eat. We also buy expensive clothes and jewelry at non-Christian retail stores because we love the things that money can buy. Most of these conferences are nothing more than a time to vacation, to glorify ourselves and some well known men of God. We leave, most of the time, with a good word that excites but has very little that is truly life changing for most of us.

The Spirit of God spoke to my heart that dedicated men and women of God longed to see more than a few manifestations of the Spirit or people jumping, shouting, and feeling glad. It seems that very few, if any, real miracles take place where many can be witnesses. In the near future, there will be conferences, not designed primarily for man's glory, but conferences that truly glorify God. These conferences will be small and will begin with from 20 to 100 people. They will have a mandatory criterion of a 7, 14 or 21-day fast prior to the conference. There will be neither food, shopping, nor patronizing during the conference. All this can be done, if possible, after the conference. These conferences will be characterized by speakers, some known, and some unknown. No matter who ministers we will only see and hear the Holy Spirit.

In our present conferences we must depend on the servant of God who is speaking to be sensitive to the Holy Spirit, or we miss what God has for us.

It is unlikely that in every conference these speakers are totally clear of mind and completely sensitive to God. In the upcoming seventh day conferences the Holy Spirit will be the focal point, and everyone unencumbered by the flesh with fasting will be sensitive to Him. Since most of these beginning conferences will be limited and closed to the public, it will be important to video tape the miraculous manifestations of God. Many people will not believe these manifestations unless they are captured on video tape. These video tapes will be shown to thousands and the Holy Spirit conferences will become larger and larger.

The Holy Spirit also revealed to me that whenever these conferences are preceded by 30 days of prayer for the city, strong principalities will be paralyzed. Pastors will also begin to call for intelligent modified fasting for weeks at a time to break the power of the enemy in their churches. Independent ministries will begin to call their staff to intelligent, modified fasting to break the power of the enemy from hindering their progress in the kingdom of God.

The Bible teaches us that at Christ's return our bodies will be translated, and will become glorified. In other words, our **triune** nature will not be necessary. We will not need to be spirit, soul and body. Our communication with God will be unencumbered by the flesh. Regular intelligent fasting causes us to know, without a doubt, God's will for our lives. When we mortify our bodies through fasting, the flesh becomes unable to hinder our understanding of the will of God. Dedicated, intelligent fasting is the closest we will ever be to a glorified body.

The Spirit of God revealed to me that there are many other well known and not so well known men and women of God who, after reading this, will confirm these words because of receiving a similar revelation from God.

Anyone can move in the power of God. Jesus said where two or three are gathered in my name, I will be there with them. The ability of the Holy Spirit is the same all the time. It is our flesh and our soulish realm that hinder us from moving and being sensitive to God. The time has come for us to take fasting to the forefront, where it needs to be. Fasting has been uncomfortable for many of us in the past, but now we can do it with fervor, allowing unencumbered communion with the Father.

Points to Remember

• Fasting is a time to learn more about God and understand yourself better. **Peter II 3:8** reveals that we are approaching the seventh day since Adam.

• We have experienced the reentrance of four major attributes into the body of Christ: justification, holiness, faith and the authority movement.

• The seventh day man (or woman) of God must embrace all four attributes. He cannot operate in one while lacking in another.

• The last two ingredients the church needed to walk in the fullness of God's purpose were the great teachers of faith and the prophetic and apolestolic enlightenment.

• When we mortify the body through fasting, the flesh is unable to hinder God's will in our lives.

• The sixth day man preached and witnessed the manifestations of the power of God, while the seventh day man will fast and see God manifest his power in a greater way to his people.

• The seventh day conferences will be an occasion to fast and pray with total focus on the Holy Spirit, unlike the sixth day conferences that center around individuals.

• Preceded by extended periods of fasting and prayer for the city, during the conferences, the principalities that rule over the city will be paralyzed.

Chapter Ten

Specifics of Fasting

Let us take a look at some specific ways to fast. Most of us don't fast very much and should begin with a one-day fast, drinking only water and juice mixed. The amount of juice should not exceed three quarter juice to one quarter steamed distilled water. Before moving on to a longer fast try the one day fast several times. This is recommended for giving the body rest and a pattern for drawing closer to God.

Fasting is not something you will do only once in a great while. It is now going to be a regular part of your Christian life. It has such benefits you will wonder why you haven't done it sooner.

Remember that fruits can be cut up and placed in a plastic bag and eaten throughout the day to curb hunger. Cereal can also be eaten with a piece of fruit and a small piece of multigrain bread. Please substitute and improvise, because it is more important to focus on God than on the specifics of what or what not to eat.

When preparing juices dilute them with 25,50 or 75% water. Thus more water is taken which is better tolerated by the stomach during a fast.

Juices should be without additives or preservatives. These can be purchased at any health food store or read the label carefully at the supermarket. Some juices labeled "pure juice" may contain sodium and other chemicals.

Since one of the main values of fasting is its cleansing ability, organic fruit should be eaten. This fruit has not been grown with chemicals or pesticides. Try not to eat more than two pieces of fruit per day on a fast. Vegetables should also be organic and about half should be eaten raw. This gives the body the benefit of the active enzymes in uncooked food

We can have water and diluted juices on demand both morning and evening. Fruits are recommended for the morning. When a person retires for the evening, he fast for 6 to 8 hours. In the morning the body needs food that can be turned without much effort into active energy. Fruits and juices can be digested in less than half an hour, thus releasing the needed energy, with less energy used by the digestive system. Vegetables and vegetable juices are good for later in the day so they are not mixed with fruits and fruit juices, as they might cause the production of unneeded gases.

Fasting has certainly changed my life and many of those around me. Most of all it has brought me closer to God and placed me in His will. I want everyone to experience the joy and excitement fasting can bring when done intelligently.

PRAYER

Dear God, I thank you for this time you have given me to minister to your people. Lord God, I ask that everyone who endeavors to fast will consult You and minister to You while on the fast. I ask that each and everyone who follows the directions on fasting understands truly what fasting is all about and will hear from You. Dear God, we know that You hear us when we minister and when we worship you. We ask that while we are on this fast You will be with us, that you will clothe us with your love, and attend to the things that plague and bother us. And that You will have an answer for every thing life presents to us. We thank you and praise you Dear God.   *Amen.*

NOTES

SUGGESTED FASTING PLANS

KEY

WATER = STEAMED DISTILLED OR FILTERED
LIQUID = DILUTED JUICES, HERBAL TEAS, WATER,
GRAIN CEREAL = OATMEAL, CREAM OF WHEAT
MALT-O-MEAL, MAPO
BREAD = MULTIGRAIN (EZEKIEL BREAD)
FRUIT = APPLES, PEARS, BANNANAS, PEACHES,
NECTARINE, GRAPES,
VEGETABLES = CABBAGE, CARROTS, ONIONS,
PEPPERS, LETTUCE, SPINACH,
SQUASH, BEANS, PEAS, ECT.

ONE DAY FAST: 24 HOURS WITH WATER ONLY

THREE DAY FAST:

DAY 1: 1 PIECE OF FRUIT IN A M
1 PIECE OF FRUIT IN P M
8-12 GLASSES OF LIQUIDS
DAY 2: 1 PIECE OF FRUIT IN A M
8-12 GLASSES OF LIQUIDS
DAY 3: 8-12 GLASSES OF WATER

SEVEN DAY FAST:

DAY 1-4: HOT GRAIN CEREAL(1 tsp. HONEY OR BROWN SUGAR), 1 SLICE MULTIGRAIN BREAD IN A M
1 PIECE OF FRUIT AT NOON
1 PIECE OF FRUIT IN P M
8-12 GLASSES OF LIQUIDS

DAY 5-6: 1 PIECE OF FRUIT IN AM
1 PIECE OF FRUIT IN P M
8-12 GLASSES OF LIQUIDS
DAY 7: 8-12 GLASSES OF WATER

TWENTY -ONE DAY FAST:

DAY 1-7: HOT GRAIN CEREAL(1 tsp. HONEY OR BROWN SUGAR), 1 SLICE MULTIGRAIN BREAD IN A M.
1 PIECE OF FRUIT AT NOON
BOWL OF RAW OR COOKED
VEGGIES IN P M
8-12 GLASSES OF LIQUIDS
DAY 8-14: HOT GRAIN CEREAL(1 tsp. HONEY OR BROWN SUGAR), 1 SLICE MULTIGRAIN BREAD IN A M.
1 PIECE OF FRUIT AT NOON
1 PIECE OF FRUIT IN P M
8-12 GLASSES OF LIQUIDS
DAY 15-18: 1 PIECE OF FRUIT IN A M
1 PIECE OF FRUIT IN P M
8-12 GLASSES OF LIQUIDS
DAY 19-20: 8-12 GLASSES OF LIQUID

DAY 21: 8-12 GLASSES OF WATER

THIRTY DAY FAST:

      DAY 1-10: HOT GRAIN CEREAL(1 tsp. HONEY OR BROWN SUGAR), AND 1 PIECE OF FRUIT, WITH 1 SLICE OF MULTIGRAIN BREAD IN A M
      1 PIECE OF FRUIT AT NOON
      BOWL OF RAW OR COOKED VEGGIES IN P M
      8-12 GLASSES OF LIQUIDS
      DAY 11-20: HOT GRAIN CEREAL(1 tsp. HONEY OR BROWN SUGAR) 1 SLICE OF MULTIGRAIN BREAD IN A M.
      1 PIECE OF FRUIT AT NOON
      BOWL OF RAW OR COOKED VEGGIES IN P M
      8-12 GLASSES OF LIQUIDS
      DAY 21-25: 1 OR 2 PIECES OF FRUIT IN A M
      1 OR 2 PIECES OF FRUIT IN P M
      8-12 GLASSES OF LIQUIDS
      DAY 26-28: 8-12 GLASSES OF LIQUIDS
      DAY 29-30: 8-12 GLASSES OF WATER

FORTY DAY FAST:

DAY 1-10: HOT GRAIN CEREAL (1 TSP.OF HONEY OR BROWN SUGAR), 1 PIECE OF FRUIT, 1 SLICE OF MULTIGRAIN BREAD IN A M
1 PIECE OF FRUIT AT NOON
BOWL OF RAW OR COOKED VEGGIES WITH 1 SLICE OF MULTIGRAIN BREAD P M
8-12 GLASSES OF LIQUIDS
DAY 11-20: HOT GRAIN CEREAL(1 tsp. HONEY OR BROWN SUGAR), 1 SLICE OF MULTIGRAIN BREAD IN A M.
1 PIECE OF FRUIT AT NOON
BOWL OF RAW OR COOKED VEGGIES IN P M .
8-12 GLASSES OF LIQUIDS
DAY 21-30: HOT GRAIN CEREAL(1 tsp. HONEY OR BROWN SUGAR), 1 SLICE OF MULTIGRAIN BREAD IN A M.
LIQUIDS AT NOON
2 PIECES FRUIT IN P M
8-12 GLASSES LIQUIDS
DAY 31-35:1 OR 2 PIECES OF FRUIT IN A M
LIQUIDS AT NOON
1 PIECE OF FRUIT IN P M
8-12 GLASSES OF LIQUIDS
DAY 36-38:8-12 GLASSES OF LIQUIDS
DAY 39-40:8-12 GLASSES OF WATER

(VITAMINS AND SUPPLEMENTS CAN BE TAKEN DAILY. THOSE ON MEDICATIONS CONSULT YOUR PHYSICIAN)

There are certainly a wide variety of things that can be consumed on a fast and varying lengths of a fasts. Please be creative as the spirit leads. The most important thing is that your relationship with GOD is improved and your ability to hear Him is enhanced.

SUGGESTIONS:

* *7 DAY LIQUID ONLY FAST FOR SPOUSE*
* *30 DAY (FRUIT & LIQIUDS DAY 1-10) FRUIT & LIQUID FAST FOR CHURCH GROWTH*
* *14 DAY LIQUID FAST FOR TEENS (DESTROY THE SPIRIT OF CONFUSION)*
* *3 DAY WATER ONLY FAST (PREPARE FOR DELIVERANCE)*
* *16 DAY (8 DAY FRUIT & LIQUID, 4 DAY LIQUID, 4 DAY WATER) FAST FOR NEW DIRECTION FOR A CHURCH*

Well , I hope that this book has certainly changed your thinking concerning fasting. I know that God will become more meaningful in your life because you will know Him better. Happy fasting and may God richly bless you.

Bibliography

Prescription for Nutritional Healing, James F Balch MD, Phyllis A. Balch, CNC Avery Publishing Group Inc. Garden City Park, NY

The Fasting Prayer, Franklin Hall

The Coming Revival, Americas call to Fast, Pray and Seek Gods face, Bill Bright, New Life Publications

Brag, Paul C. and Patricia, The Miracle of Fasting (Santa Barbara CA: Health Science, n. d.)

Prince, Derek. Fasting (Springdale, PA: Whitaker House 1986)

Foster, Richard J., Celebration of Discipline (San Francisco : Harper - San Francisco, 1988)

Chatham , R. D. , Fasting: A Biblical- Historical Study (South Plainfield, NJ : Bridge Publishing, 1987)

If My People, by Sun Fannin , Companion Press 1992

Seductions Exposed, The Spiritual Dynamics of Relationships Dr. Gary L Greenwald, (Eagles Nest Publications Santa Ana, CA)